Cradle of Heaven

The arms of the mother are the cradle of heaven . . .

— Hazrat Inayat Khan

Cradle of Heaven

Psychological and Spiritual Dimensions of Conception, Pregnancy, and Birth

Murshida Vera Justin Corda

Omega
Press

Lebanon Springs, New York

3/95

Cradle of Heaven: Psychological and Spiritual Dimensions of
Conception, Pregnancy, and Birth
© 1987 by Vera Justin Corda. All rights reserved.
10 9 8 7 6 5 4 3 2 1

Omega Press
P.O. Box 574
Lebanon Springs, New York 12114

Library of Congress Catalog Card No. 87-061934

Printed in the United States of America
ISBN 0-930872-32-0

Dedication

To the love children of the eighties whose quality of soul, far outreaching our own, will enable them to build the bridges of peace and brotherhood we laid the foundations for and to their guides, parents, and teachers who will unlearn and learn again from them.

Contents

Foreword

Perhaps one of the greatest needs of our time is for the re-spiritualization of life. This does not mean the superimposition of "spiritual value" upon the world but in its simplest and perhaps most profound form, it refers to an appreciation of life as inherently spiritual. In this light, what can be a more profound experience than conception and childbirth — the bringing forth of new life into the world? But unfortunately our western approaches have made childbirth so "natural" and sterilized as to effectively de-sanctify this most significant rite of the human passage. Long overdue is a re-sanctification of the birthing process through the contemplation, with awe, of its mystery and meaning.

In this book, Vera Corda has done a magnificent job of returning this auspicious occasion to its rightful context as a sacred experience. Health and spirituality are reunited in a highly informative, practical, and moving work that will be of immense benefit to mothers, fathers, families, and all caretakers and attendants of the cradle of heaven.

Lawrence M. Spiro, Ph.D.
Founder, *Melia Foundation*

Author's Preface

Mothering seems to have gone awry in our fast-moving civilization that appears to have bypassed intuition of the heart. We have forgotten what our pioneer forefathers and foremothers took for granted in infant care before the pediatric profession came into being. In the West, we have lost the art of nurturing the birthing mother, ourselves, and our men. Somehow we must return to natural, intuitive ways, for when a civilization becomes too mental, as is the trend today, it will destroy itself.

One purpose of this book is to help caretakers develop the ability to attune to their children through observing what is happening in their five developmental bodies: physical, mental, emotional, spiritual, and ethical/moral, regardless of their chronological age. There are some skills and knowledge that our culture does not pass on, perhaps due to the waning focus on family nurturance, directly reflected in the increasing number of single-parent families in our fast-changing society. Motherhood and fatherhood consist of a series of skills we relearn in life's greatest challenge — parenting.

Postbirth energy is usually centered on the infant's care, but in older societies, postbirth care included brushing the mother's hair, sponge-bathing her, massaging her arms, and giving her loving embraces. Today birthing coaches, midwives, and close friends of the couple who attend the birth take over this function. Caring gestures are as important as good nutrition and should be encouraged by this support group, for it will be modeling the caregiving skills the mother will soon use in her own nurturing.

Most of our fathers had little or no role in our delivery, other than getting our mothers to the hospital. Planting of the seed seemed to conclude his part of conception until a bundle was placed in his arms hours or even days after its birth. Excluded from the birthing scene, he missed those crucial first moments when the soul enters this life on the breath. Hospital rules allowed no immediate eye contact with his own infant. The euphoria passed and all too soon the father returned to his lonely home, feeling separation, strangeness, and sometimes even estrangement from his wife and his child.

New age couples emerging from the culture of the late sixties and seventies felt it vitally important that the father be reinstated in his rightful place as the birthing coach and assistant, whereas previously they might have chosen to allow the physician and hospital staff almost full responsibility for birthing their child. In a society striving to establish equal rights for men and women, it is strange that in most hospitals today fathers do not have equal rights with mothers in bonding to their children in the birthing room. Home births have changed this practice.

Another purpose of this book is to fill in empty spots in understanding the complex role of parenting today. Bonding with the new soul enables us to unlearn and relearn at every level. Only through reliving our childhood by growing up again with our children — adopted, foster, or those we guide — can we be made whole and complete in our own development. Living experience, backed by peer-group sharing, builds parenting skills and self-confidence. Parents can also learn from mother nature and the way she shares her bounty with us, regardless of whether we are deserving or not. The most important role that parents and caretakers can play in children's development is to provide an environment of unconditional love in which children can learn about our world. Love, not "things," builds that kind of atmosphere.

Acknowledgments

No book is ever written alone and this one owes much to the many who contributed their time and energy. To Pir Vilayat Khan, my teacher and guide; to the committee that saw that this book reached you — Richard Page, Dr. Leonard Levis, Mary Lee Levis, and particularly, Zahira Marla Rabinowitz, who edited the manuscript and coordinated production; to Norman Kanter, who designed the book cover; to Mary Crawford, who painstakingly copied my illustrations; to Matina Kilkenny and Aeolea Ray, who proofread the final manuscripts; to John Futhey for his contribution of computer equipment and expertise; to Robin Collier for his invaluable assistance in the final stages of production; and to my devoted helpmeet, James Corda, who kept the home fires burning through it all. I am deeply appreciative of their encouragement and loving labor.

To the thirty-seven infants of the Marin Infancy School in San Rafael, California and to their parents and aides, whose observation and care gave inspiration and validity to this work.

To the mothers and fathers all over the United States and the world who gave support and friendship in thousands of letters that passed between us over the years. To the Hawaiian mothers and fathers who contributed so much to the waterbirth chapter. To the mothers and fathers of our community whose involvement and feedback kept me going.

To Esther Thompson, from the Marin Nursing Association, who encouraged and gave unstintingly of her counsel to the Marin Infancy School.

To the believers in the message for children over the years

whose financial backing made this first edition possible and whose names are too myriad to mention, thank you dear brothers and sisters.

Last but not least, to Patricia Walia Laszewski, whose direction and record-keeping at the Marin Infancy Center provided the heart and courage to carry it all to completion.

Thank you, Beloved Ones.

About the Author

Murshida Vera Corda has devoted her life to her work as an educator and spiritual counselor. Through successful careers in ballet, graphic arts design, nursing, and teaching, she has, over the last forty years, gained recognition as an expert in early childhood education and family development and as a spiritual guide to parents and children.

Beginning her training in the care and education of young children at the age of ten at the innovative Canon Kip Nursery School in the south-of-Market area of San Francisco, she went on to receive an Associate's degree in the field of graphic arts at the age of sixteen. She later received a Bachelor of Arts degree in education and completed a Master of Arts degree in the education of exceptional children at the University of California at San Francisco. While receiving additional training at Columbia University she studied with the leading pediatric expert, Arnold Gesell. She is currently a Joel Katz Memorial Scholar, earning a Ph.D. degree in guidance and counseling at Columbia Pacific University.

Murshida Vera taught in the public schools for fifteen years and holds a lifetime teacher's credential in California. Early in her career she worked at the San Francisco Youth Guidance Center and at Langley Porter Neuropsychiatric Institute employing art therapy principles and techniques with disturbed youth. Through a variety of WPA programs and projects, she began establishing nursery schools where she trained parents and childcare directors in child and family guidance. She is also a registered nurse and practiced psychiatric nursing at Dewitt

State Hospital in California.

Murshida Vera Corda has been a practicing Sufi disciple for over fifty years and was given the title of Murshida, or spiritual teacher, many years ago when she began guiding other disciples in the Sufi tradition. During the early seventies she founded the New Age Seed Schools in the San Francisco Bay Area, based in the studies and teachings of the Sufi master, Hazrat Inayat Khan. She developed a complete curriculum from infancy through elementary school and trained teachers and parents in the spiritual, intellectual, social, physical, and moral development of children.

For the past twenty years she has been a practicing healer in the Sufi Order, the Sufi Islamia Ruhaniat Society, and the Order of St. Luke. Murshida Vera Corda continues to tutor children with special learning needs at her home in the Salinas Valley and travels throughout the United States guiding people in their spiritual pursuits, teaching spiritual healing and development, leading individual and group retreats, and training parents and educators in the guidance of children from preconception through adolescence.

Introduction

As one looks at the life cycle it becomes apparent that there are critical events that are of profound significance in their ability to influence human development. The transition to parenthood is perhaps the most remarkable of all life's developmental stages. Successful completion of the tasks accompanying the transition has the most important influence on family functioning. Profound implications for psychological and spiritual growth are inherent in the transformation from an identity as a couple to an identity as a family. The manner in which this phase of development is negotiated by its participants is thought to lay the foundation for the psychological and emotional well-being of each family member. Patterns for the handling of individual and family needs for dependency, nurturance, growth, and autonomy may become firmly established during this transition. As a couple adjusts to the arrival of the newborn, levels of intimacy between partners may be challenged and a deepened awareness of each one's capacity for commitment realized.

Pregnancy is a time of turning inward, when one's sense of purpose may be expanded, when one's awareness of the mystery of life may become heightened, and when one may open one's soul to honest examination. It is also a time when religious and spiritual concerns may naturally arise and the incorporation of spiritual practices into one's life may take on new importance and meaning. It is no wonder that the psychological literature has often referred to this period as a developmental crisis.

Over the past fifteen to twenty years there has been a

growing interest among professionals and parents in gaining an understanding of the psychological experience of pregnancy. Prior to this time, most literature on pregnancy emphasized fetal development and focused on guiding parents on proper pre-natal care. Little attention was paid to the psychological and emotional impact of pregnancy and childbirth on the parents. Early psychological research in child development focused pri-marily on descriptions of the various stages of a child's cogni-tive, emotional, and social development and on the impact of various parenting styles and practices, particularly mothering, on the child's later development. Even less attention was paid to the influence of fathering on the child's development. Most early investigations of fathering focused on the impact of "father absence" on the child's development. Only recently, as parents have begun to expand upon traditional roles, a body of litera-ture has emerged that begins to describe the important and unique aspects of the father-infant relationship. Unfortunately, as in the case of mothers, much of that research has overlooked the impact of the father's involvement in early parenting on his own development and view of himself.

In those early years of research the reciprocal influences in-herent in family and individual development were largely overlooked. That is, the influence of the child's developmental changes on the parent's growth and functioning was beyond the scope of most studies. Currently, a model of research and theory of development that recognizes the truly interactive na-ture of human development has become popular. Researchers are increasing their attempts to capture and describe human development from a family developmental perspective. Many recent studies focus on normal transitions in the family life cy-cle and view the changing nature of individual needs in the context of relationships to significant others in the family.

The growth of the alternative birth movement, the surge of interest in shared conscious parenting, and the gradual change in birthing practices to involve the father in a meaningful way have all contributed to a new perspective on pregnancy and birth. This impetus has led researchers, professionals, and parents to consider the many aspects of the transition to parenthood in more depth and with more respect for its complexities.

What is being discovered is that the consolidation of one's identity as a parent is a complex developmental process that does not begin with the birth of the child, but begins much earlier, even before conception. As young children, we play at being parents, internalizing models and images from our own parents. As adults we may imagine what it would be like to have a child and how we would like to overcome the perceived limitations of our own upbringing. But despite the level of inner preparedness one may bring to parenthood, the onset of pregnancy and the anticipation of the birth awakens a developmental surge of tremendous proportion. The archetypal "parent within" is activated and comes alive. Many prospective parents report that concerns in both the inner and outer realms come to the fore with a new sense of urgency. Typically, parents describe a sorting out process in which the unresolved issues in their personal development press for deep consideration and resolution. Values and priorities are questioned and clarified, and childhood experiences with their own parents are reappraised. This reappraisal of the past provides an opportunity for reconciliation with the events of childhood as parenting is approached with a new level of understanding. In this light, as prospective parents are reawakened to all aspects of their heritage, issues from their religious and spiritual upbringing may be reevaluated.

We are presently witnessing a growing widespread interest in and commitment to spiritual growth and development. The reasons for this are varied and numerous, but it is clear that there is an emerging consciousness and recognition among many individuals of a need to define life experiences in spiritual terms. Particularly in our highly technological society, where external, visible accomplishments are highly valued and our cultural orientation is largely towards the outer world, we have seen a growing awareness of the need for inner accomplishment and the development of the inner being. Many have turned to the spiritual paths of the East and Eastern mysticism to find this balance. Deeply valued and respected in the traditions of the East, the inner journey has now found a place in Western society.

Many who are choosing this path express that the greatest challenge is to incorporate their spiritual practice and concentration into everyday life. The desire is not to withdraw from the world but rather to discover the spiritual element in relation to the world. In this context, it is natural that we should begin to look to such important events as pregnancy and the transition to parenthood for their potential enhancement of spiritual and emotional growth. Further, it is appropriate that the total family be the focus of spiritual and psychological study.

The commitment to gaining an increased consciousness about life through spiritual practice and psychological self-examination has captured the interest of many, including parents, therapists, counselors, childbirth educators, family practitioners, and others who work with expectant parents. Murshida Vera Corda is a highly respected educator, counselor, and spiritual guide in the Sufi tradition. Her work is nonsectarian. It represents a fresh new approach to the transition to parenthood and the experience of parenting. It relates the spiritual path to normal developmental events in a way that enables the individual to integrate spirituality in the home. *Cradle of Heaven* offers parents and professionals a new vision of how to make spirituality a vital part of becoming a family. This book is a guide, presented in a manner that does not draw sharp distinctions between religious orientations. Rather, it seeks to transcend these differences and is purely spiritual in nature and intent. Murshida Vera's work extends the psychological aspects of pregnancy, childbirth, and the transition to parenthood into the spiritual realm.

Leonard Levis, Ph.D.
Clinical Director, *West Coast Children's Center*
Albany, California

CHAPTER ONE

Conception

Just as the image of the full-blown rose cannot be imagined in the tight green bud; as the miracle of the baby at birth cannot be imagined to grow from the microscopic union of sperm and egg; conception remains a sacred and beautiful mystery. The mystery of conception awes and subtly leads to higher spiritual attunement between man and woman, while stimulating the search for deeper understanding of the purpose of life. This same act of divine creation within humankind has been occurring for eons, yet to each couple who fully experiences the miracle of union, it is like again becoming the first parents in the garden of Eden. The male and female energies meet, recreating the entire evolution of mankind in the microcosm of the woman's womb — ever a miracle, in any place or time. In celebration of this recurring awesome event, ancient peoples deified the Great Mother. Examples are seen in clay figurines of the Mother Goddess in North Baluchistan, India; the Venus of Willendorf, Germany; Isis in Egypt; Mary in Nazareth; Kwan Yin in China and Tibet; and Shakti in India.[1] Each woman, in reenacting that mystery, becomes the Divine Mother, a being she discovers within her own nature.

CONCEPTION AS SPIRITUAL INITIATION FOR WOMEN

The man, passing his sperm with intent to conceive his child, transfers with will the roots of his heritage into another generation — immortality in the flesh. In accepting his mate as an aspect of the Divine Mother, he also partakes of a spiritual reenactment of his own adoration of the female principle. For the male, conception is emotionally a rite of passage, since the act of releasing sperm is transported from being merely an experience of thrilling relief to realization of his divine purpose in mature manhood. No longer can his ego stand self-enclosed; from this moment on, a part of his inviolate self has been released willingly into another entity. His seed growing within another being spiritually expands his consciousness, readying him for the miracle of birth and acceptance of his child as an extension of himself.

The desire to love and be loved may lure men and women into few or many relationships, one of which, through conception, may awaken the woman to the selfless, loving service of motherhood. Motherhood is one of the highest spiritual initiations a woman receives on this earth plane. However, to understand this initiation, one must understand more about initiations throughout life. Birth in itself initiates infants into the mystery of life and breath. As infants cut their first molars, self-will begins. The day infants stand on their own feet and become toddlers, free to move at will; to stand, no longer crawling upon the earth; free of the parents' supporting arms, they have been initiated into a new space and dimension. With discovery of the erogenous zones — the clitoris or penis — followed by the desire to kiss little boys or girls, comes the first realization that the sexual anatomy is designed for a purpose.

At nine years of age another initiation takes place: the child reaches a mental plateau from which is distilled an understanding of what has been modeled these past nine years. An inner evaluation occurs, a milestone on the way to puberty.

The next initiation takes place when the child confronts her own sexual needs and gratifications for the first time. With this experience comes the first inner judgment of goodness versus badness, self-gratification versus renunciation; this is followed by confrontation with an inner guide. Often forgotten, this experience is reencountered during the birthing experience with new understanding. When menarche (the onset of menstruation) is reached, the initiation into womanhood brings into a girl's consciousness her divine destiny as the protector and sustainer of the race. The test of her womanhood is yet to come. The search for personal love begins.

As with all spiritual initiations (save menarche), conception is preceded by a test. For each woman, the hours of knowing she has or may have conceived are likely to be emotionally charged and full of mental turmoil. The woman may not have yet missed her period when this begins. The nature of the test is that it requires the woman to become receptive to the unknown: the unknown child, the unknown skills and understanding, the unknown woman she will become. If a woman opens up to this growth and trusts herself, she will pass through the initial crisis of doubt and fear that seems to beset even the most maternal of women.

The very nature of testing depends upon the experience of life. Life itself is the test and there is no end to the testing as long as the person breathes. Each experience is a confrontation with a new aspect of the totality of being: for the expectant mother, a new relationship between herself and the fetus — with the placenta being the medium of physical exchange. Mentally, the father relates to the child through the mother. The testing manifests in the mental attitude of the new mother, which swings as a pendulum from joy to fearfulness of her own inadequacy — to facing the new responsibility with renewed expectation.

Conception is initially a crisis due to the nature of this testing. It is an inner battle to give up being master of her own body to the domination of the developing fetus, with its needs and demands. The crisis of pregnancy, then, is that turning point in a woman's life in which she stands apart from her old single-minded self to become the servant of and first guide to the incoming soul. The mental acceptance by the father and the spiritual acceptance by the mother determine the power and duration of this time of crisis. The crisis demands that she understand exactly what commitment to motherhood means to her particular lifestyle. During this test, reactions to former crises in her life cannot be used as models nor are they useful for assurance. Her mate can best give the backup and encouragement needed during the first days of pregnancy. Gradually, the integration of self-love and love for the new entity occurs and this phase melts away into a feeling of joyous fulfillment. The single mother will need a dear friend and counselor in lieu of the husband-father.

Working through the test successfully requires many changes in thinking. Conception is a positive occurrence because it forces the woman to grow and learn anew through the expansion of her consciousness. Most changes in her life have come in spite of herself. In mentally accepting this most divine of life's experiences, either by an act of God or through her own willfulness, the transformation takes place.

Change becomes a chain reaction. Each change in environment brings about new relationships. New relationships change personal goals and objectives and demand growth in new areas of our beings. It is this enforced growth in consciousness through physical experience that tests her character to its foundations. Out of the depths of her heart, former experiences are recalled and reevaluated with regard to the present experience. The expansion of her consciousness frees her for taking on new responsibilities and expanding her outlook on her future life as mother and mate.

She can begin to comprehend that conception awakens her to the real purpose of her womanhood. What is the purpose of life — to learn; to be fulfilled; to be of service; to guide another? Until the time of pregnancy, a woman's entire lifestyle is self-planned and she merely goes with the flow of life. Suddenly this new being invades her body, forcing her to listen to a new rhythm and to give in to a will stronger than her own. She soon learns that the old self-image does not fit that which impending motherhood demands. She must eat for two, rest or be kicked into listening by her nerves and muscles, control her breath or be controlled by her emotions. The growing fetus becomes an unbidden, everpresent teacher who demands listening to a new body language. She learns that pride in her lithe, free body must become pride in a strange new profile. People she meets in markets or shops begin to aid her, each unknowingly assisting in the transition toward a self-image that embraces her new and beautiful motherhood. The word "madonna" takes on new meaning as strangers' eyes light up at the sight of her growing tummy. The protection and caring she receives from mate and friends at first may embarrass or frustrate her, until she learns to accept them. Gradually and quite subtly, the entity within her can change her whole outlook on the meaning of roots, family, and a nest.

The awe that comes with the new responsibility for another soul often grows into realization of what it really means to be a woman. The changes in her mate's and her own roles may develop new understanding of her desire to serve the needs of another in a loving way. All children often catch the pregnant woman's eye and touch her heart, awakening the desire to protect, to guide, and to nurture all helpless young. She may begin to understand the universal mothers of the world — childless women who mother other people's children. These great mothers and most saintly souls, the Mother Theresas of the world, often attract her attention and become her inspiration. As she reads and contemplates their mothering instinct, her own often becomes stronger in order to prepare her to serve her own child. All children may potentially become her children; all suffering of the young may feel as though it were hers to allay; all needs of innocent beings may become her concern. The mothering instinct often awakens from her heart's need to serve.

In understanding life, she may find that life gives her fulfillment only as she is willing to relinquish her self-will. In exchange, new privileges often come as grace — blessings not earned but falling as "gentle rain falls from heaven." The appreciation of her own parents often blossoms at this time. She may remind herself that although parents are given the gift of a child to enjoy, love, and nurture, this child does not belong to her or her mate; the infant is a child of God loaned to them. In facing the pure light and innocence of her friends' newborn babies and those infants she sees on the streets, the great privilege and responsibility of parenthood may confront her. Both parents-to-be may suddenly see the world full of pregnant women and babies and feel the awe of new life.

There can be fulfillment in passing through all the stages of growth with her child. She may remember or relearn each corresponding stage in her own life, possibly completing phases of development left unfinished due to emotional trauma or illness. The father, too, may experience this completion to a greater or lesser degree, depending upon his bonding with the incoming soul.

The precious and sacred work of bringing life into the world helps the woman see herself as divine. If she has had not only the experience of birthing her own child, but of saving a life, of being a foster or adopted parent to her mate's child(ren), or of giving life and protection to the motherless beings not born from her own body, she has inherited fulfillment. The reward for losing self in the loving service to another's child is the ability to realize and manifest one's higher self.

Even as life gives fulfillment, so it calls for responsibility and service from a woman to teach, guide, nurture, and protect the young. Conception brings upon women and men a facing-up to adult responsibilities, a rite of passage into maturity that eventually transforms the independent, indifferent being into the self-sacrificing guide of another soul. Part of this new understanding about the purpose of womanhood brings not only acceptance of life, but acceptance of its counterpart, death. New life on this plane means a kind of death on a former plane. Pregnancy can encourage a woman to face the death of her old self; in the passage to the new self she understands the sacredness of giving life — the mystery of pregnancy and birth — the rite of becoming a mother.

Leaving behind the old self and stretching her consciousness to accommodate another being will, indeed, develop selflessness and renunciation. Now she realizes that her initial fear of pregnancy was really fear of losing her freedom. In truth, only the lesser self is lost in motherhood. Attention to the fetus developing within her and attuning to the nature of that being can shrink all thought of the limited self. The feeling that her body is expanding outward to accommodate the child is put into perspective by perceiving that the outer universe exists within herself. The greater Self is being realized. Forgetting self can pave the way for a great and abiding happiness to enter her consciousness. Renunciation of personal freedom, which at first may frighten and then may challenge her to the depths of her being, is now understood. Former goals and objectives, once held so dear, can be subjugated to the urgency of procreation and then the demanding role of guide.

In becoming a nurturing mother who helps establish firm psychological, physical, mental, spiritual, and social foundations in her child, she will be challenged to relinquish her personal goals for at least the first two-and-a-half years. This is the time when the mold of character and personality takes place. The ancient wisdom ascribing total impressionability to the newborn soul has been corroborated by recent research. Under hypnosis, children have accurately described their birth experiences in great detail (as compared with the description by their mothers, also under hypnosis). The recollections were so vivid that conversations, physical appearances, methods of delivery, and emotional states of mother, father, doctor, and nurse were all noted.[2]

The subconscious mind is a reservoir of all experiences; early life experiences form the vessel in which later experiences will be contained. The pregnant woman may take this realization into her heart and strive to create a beneficial environment for the new soul's unfoldment. She may feel no sacrifice can be too great during these first years of mother-impress on her child. She may be willing to give up habits of personal gratification (such as drinking alcohol, smoking tobacco or marijuana, taking any type of drug, or eating obsessively) that injure the developing fetus.[3,4] The island of security built around the self must be slowly washed away in the waters of life. For the single woman, these self-denials may seem to be more difficult without the father's backup. The sacrifices the single woman makes, even unwillingly, when she accepts her pregnancy, are an example of diving deep into Self and finding unity with a force greater than herself. This enables her to accept more responsibility than she had believed she was capable of. A key aspect of motherhood is the constant testing of patience. Initially, a woman has little choice. She must wait patiently for nine months while her child develops within her. Pregnancy is a time of waiting that builds tolerance for the daily patience required in mothering. The patience she learns during her days in waiting eventually gives a peace and inner security in the divine mission of procreation. Graciously, God has built into growth a pendulum that swings from high achievement to low plateaus, where little or nothing, save the passing of time, seems to be happening. Calm endurance of the physical discomfort and rampant curiosity in the last weeks of pregnancy teach the essential lesson that prepares a mother to stand the daily grind of caretaking.

Conception is a test that requires a woman's self-image to grow. Her concept of her own destiny as well as her girlhood dreams and ambitions are shaken. Holding onto a rapidly vanishing limited version of herself becomes increasingly difficult. If a good mother image is not within the woman's own life experience, the fearful determination to become a good mother will need much reinforcement by her mate or, if she is a single woman, by her close friends. She will need reassurance that women are not born mothers but learn caretaking skills through observation of peers, personal experience, and love.

We presume that every woman is born with the ability to nurture her young. This is not necessarily true. In our increasingly isolated nuclear families, many women have never handled a baby until the birth of their own. In contrast, in South and Central American families, every little girl witnesses and participates in the care of siblings. She has learned long before the birth of her own child the meanings of the different cries of the infant, when to pick it up and when to leave it to its own company, and how to pacify, care for, and nurture the infant. This enables a young girl to attune to mothering in a confident manner long before she becomes a mother. She models her own mother's child-rearing practices. If her own parents separated before she reached eleven years of age, she often has problems in the early care of her own child.[5]

Making the changes necessary for motherhood can be a challenge to the woman, particularly if her early foundation in nurturance is weak. Change is always difficult, but it is the everpresent goal in life. New or borrowed maternity clothes, a new nest, new friendships with other pregnant women, and the ensuing exchange of dreams and plans for parenting pave the way toward transformation of her self-image.

Some women find it trying to give up their careers. They may be emotionally and financially stable, with a mature mate relationship and well-developed ideas for being a mother, yet the care and nurturance of the child alone does not seem to be fulfilling enough. Ideally, the child needs the first two-and-a-half years of the mother's total devotion and concentration before the mother resumes a former out-of-the-home career. This is not to say that the mother cannot develop herself during this period, making time for her own interests and undertaking some activities that relate to her career goals. However, her complete centering on the child during this time makes the difference in all later transitions and developmental crises.

Many women experience a feeling of psychological unreadiness to take total responsibility for another soul. Leah, in her early twenties, described her reaction to conception.

> I didn't think I could cope or was ready for this responsibility. I wanted to finish school, and our finances were extremely tight. I became deeply depressed and considered abortion several times, even to the point of making an ap-

pointment. My husband was loving and supportive and said that without a doubt he wanted to be a father, but if I felt I couldn't handle it he would support my decision. Soon I knew that there was no way in the world I could have had an abortion. It would have been a tragedy for both of us. As soon as I mentally accepted the challenge of motherhood, the accommodation began. The mother image melded over me like a veil that could not again be taken off. I then felt divinely gifted, honored to be the vessel for this new life. The only important thing was preparing for this child. Never in my life had I been so totally centered around one thing.

In the early days and weeks following conception it may be helpful for the woman to get psychological counseling if the inner battle is too disturbing to resolve itself or if the partner is unsupportive.

CONCEPTION AS SPIRITUAL INITIATION FOR MEN

The prospective father also goes through a crisis. Conception is a rite of passage for him, too, as well as an opportunity to grow spiritually and mentally. The whole chain of consequences that follows conception forces the man to come to terms with his spiritual goals and objectives. There is a dramatic change in his emotional body and in the quality of the relationship with his mate. Acceptance of fatherhood changes his perspective on life. The responsibility of providing for his enlarged family forces him to reevaluate his own qualities and capacities. How shall he extend his studies? Should he change jobs or seek advancement where he now works? He mulls matters over and changes his mind often. He tells himself that he must now change his self-image from a carefree, independent being to a responsible parent. Preparation for being a model for his child's learning about masculinity challenges his higher self. He wishes to support his mate in her new role as the mother of his child, while at the same time feeling a need for support himself. Frequently, his desire is to be both spiritual support and mental comforter as well as best friend, amateur masseur and mature lover.

Sex and parenting should always go hand in hand. When responsibility is taken for the possibility of conception in the sexual act, the mate can aid the woman greatly in accepting her mothering role, for all women do not willingly open themselves to conception. In some relationships, the woman's rejection of even the idea of conceiving children can collapse the man's self-image. The play of insecurities can be debilitating. Conversely, for the man, a relationship with a woman who has a positive attitude toward becoming a mother can be a key that opens him to the fathering role. Mutual support is needed.

The man who fails to take responsibility for conception is not aware of his behavior in relation to his subconscious mind. His whole self is involved in the sexual act, so it follows that this most sacred act demands total absorption by his whole being. Consciously creating a new life culminates in full realization of manhood.

Mentally, each woman must accept her pregnancy by free choice. The way in which she passes through the crisis of indecision will forever affect her attitude toward the male ego, her future love relationships, and her own self-image. When the mother-to-be is reinforced positively by an emotionally ready father-to-be, her role as sweetheart is easily transformed into the first guide of her child. Her boy-lover, like the frog prince of fairy tales, transforms himself into the new and important image of protector, provider, and reinforcing second guide to her child and herself. Parenting is accepted as the inevitable fulfillment of this greatest of all rites of passage, as a sacred trust to guide and nurture an emerging soul into the physical vehicle created by an act of love between two people.

Many strong and erratic changes take place in the mother during the transition. A change in lifestyle takes place as her body demands to be heard. A change in her relationship with the child's father takes place as she begins seeing him in a new role. At last, a great joy can flood her heart and mind through realization of her womanhood. The man, too, can come through the period of self-inquiry and realize his readiness for fatherhood as well as the continued growth that he and his mate will share together as parents.

THE SOUL'S JOURNEY TO EARTH

For the incoming soul, conception also leads to spiritual attunement and deeper existential understanding. Conception for the soul is an initiation preceded by a test, which is the long spiritual journey to the earth that begins in the angelic spheres. "Every soul is an angel before it touches the earth," explained the Sufi master, Inayat Khan.[6] The qualities of this sphere are unlike those of the earth plane, with its desires that, in most cases, mute the innocence and simplicity of the angelic being. The angelic kingdom is free from distinctions that human minds insist upon making. Divine love and unity are the qualities that pervade this sphere, even though the essence of individual personality is inherent in each angelic soul. The soul, here as elsewhere, is creative, and the angelic soul has intelligence — it lives in a purely mental world, a world created by thought-form alone. Each soul lives as an electrical current, an energy force beyond space and time. It is entranced into the body by the love experience of its parents.

The soul, being a luminescent electromagnetic force, travels on the divine sun's rays. Each soul is cast forth into the manifestation that each ray describes. While descending to the earth, the soul emerges into the djinn, or genius plane, where mind and soul unite with intuition and inspiration to produce the spirit. In Sanskrit, genius means "knowledge," or "jnana." Not until life on earth begins will the mind be completed. "The soul on its journey from the unseen to the seen world receives impressions from the souls which are on their return journey from the seen to the unseen. In this way, the soul collects the first merits, qualities, and sometimes, limitations, which discipline its field of action. It is this which forms a pathway for the soul to follow, and it is this pathway that leads it to the parents from whom it inherits its later attributes."[7] Since the soul is creative in essence it cannot help being impressed by great souls that have remained on the djinn plane to assure that their incomplete earth work is carried forward for the benefit of humanity. Thus, the inspirations of geniuses have extended the consciousness of mankind through invention, art, science, and social progress. Not all impress on the djinn plane is that of the "genius" (as we interpret it in English). Souls going home do, however, linger and give their impress to angels coming into manifestation, in order to see their interrupted work carried forward on earth and also to strengthen the incoming souls for the shock of our plane.

SOULS WANT EMBODIMENT

Souls, anxious for embodiment after dwelling in the djinn plane, often hover and annoy couples in bed until they are conceived. Particularly during times of great devastation, many souls are forced out of their bodies against their will: especially during famines, wars, explosions, floods, earthquakes, and other disasters. Many souls are waiting to be reincarnated, persistently struggling for embodiment — sometimes, in their eagerness, preventing their earth parents from the normal fulfillment of their life goals. At this moment, every day, in different parts of the world, there are many deaths that we have little awareness of. There are thousands of souls being knocked out of their bodies suddenly, without warning or expectation, as opposed to dying from diseased conditions or old age. When death is unexpected and unaccepted, it thrusts that entity, without its will or knowledge, into the astral plane and this causes the soul to be what is called "earthbound." The desire of earthbound souls to come back into the body is very strong. These are the souls that hover around without being called in on the love wave. Parents' matings are not trying to attract them because the prospective parents do not feel that this is particularly the time when they want to welcome a child into their family. Yet here are all these souls — hovering and waiting — anxious to be born again in order to fulfill their soul goals.

This phenomenon occurs in waves. At all periods in history there have been souls trying to complete a life experience — and not always where they are welcomed. Their urgency is related to the period of time that they can stay earthbound, for if they do not find reembodiment within a certain period, they must go on; the cycle turns and they are put into other planes where they do not have that chance again. So they battle and fight to get through, using every and any trickery or method that will allow them to manifest.

Sometimes the soul makes itself known to one or both of the lovers by manifesting through sight, sound, scent, dreams, intuition, or feelings. The soul usually comes quite unbidden by the couple to announce its choice of the parents it needs to fulfill its life purpose. The hovering soul, hungry for embodiment, is held captive over the mother's navel. At birth, with the first breath the infant takes, the soul will enter the baby. The soul's determination to embody and its persistent appearances amaze the couple whose collective mind is often set in opposition to the new soul's efforts, which sometimes drive the male from his marriage bed to postpone an uninvited conception.

Here is one such experience.

John and Rose had joyfully welcomed the birth of their first three children but now felt they had all the family they could support and educate. Despite their mutual agreement on this point and their faithfulness in practicing contraceptive methods, John had a recurring unusual experience. It seemed that on every new moon he would feel a presence in their room and when he listened intently and sought to explain it, with his night sight he would see little round lights, about the size of ping-pong balls, with fluttering wings, dancing around their bed. Recognizing this phenomena intuitively as souls seeking embodiment in a loving environment, he accused Rose of seeking secretly for another pregnancy. She emphatically denied this. In desperation, he would leave his bed to sleep in another room. Rose anxiously sent out thought forms: "Go away, we do not want to parent you. Find someone else." She added a third method of contraception to the two she already was practicing faithfully. The little lights disappeared and John once more occupied his bed with Rose. Then one night in her safe time and with all precautions taken, a little light danced in anyway! "I still don't know how this could be!" Rose told me, "but we certainly have a fourth child to prove it."

A younger woman in her twenties, Stephanie, wrote of her conception experience:

This particular night was the night Greg and I decided to be married — nothing could keep us apart. Before either one of us came to orgasm, I began feeling like I was conceiving, or had conceived, or was going to conceive — an overwhelming compulsion that I had no control over, the first real understanding of what making love was all about. We climaxed together, coming into a very high place. Totally worn out, we lay there in impenetrable peace and stillness.

Through the open window above us, a puff of summer wind scented with jasmine and sweet blossoms, laden with the summer life force, moved the curtains and flowed down over us like liquid air. The candle began fluttering in a strange way. The room was dense with an unseen presence — air so thick I hardly dared breathe. We lay there with eyes wide open, our spines tingling, expecting a manifestation. But this soul was intangible — felt, yet unseen. Yes, I did conceive!

Occasionally, conception is a spiritual experience much like inner initiation for the woman. Here is a conception experience excerpted from one woman's spiritual journal.

This night in meditation I beheld the sun at the dawn of

creation. A ray shot forth, swift as an arrow, straight and true, shattering the "I" of me and the will of my beloved mate. Engulfed, flooded, lifted on spiraled sound — oh cherubim and serafim, your song enchanted one soul and, in its ecstasy, angel became djinn within me. Oh Divine Mother, in sweet passivity enfold myself in Thy mantle that I may bring forth a perfect child.

The author recalls her first experience with conception, as a child.

My younger sister was ten years old and I eleven, when my mother, to her consternation, conceived. She was beginning menopause at the time. When forced to admit to her lady friends at almost six months along that she was, indeed, pregnant, she would hastily add, "by accident." This was in the 1920s — a time of change for women — when bobbed hair, flapper clothes, and bathtub gin were prevalent, yet many women's awareness of their sexuality was still fraught with misunderstanding and Victorian modesty.

Such a great event in our lives was not to be announced to us children by Mama, although we questioned between us what was wrong with her, since she cried often in the locked bathroom to Daddy. It was my maternal grandmother who was finally given the job of "explaining it to the children." I can't say I was surprised. Hadn't I seen her cherub's face flying around my parent's bed? Today, many parents tell me that an older child knew of the pregnancy and the sex of the child before the couple had any idea that they were pregnant. Siblings' love attracts souls too.

Months later, the baby arrived and was sent to live with my mother's mother in an adjoining flat. Mother continued her life unencumbered, save for strictly scheduled nursing times. The baby was mine, however, every Saturday morning, when I was allowed to ride her around our block in her pram.

Years later, my mother told me that she simply could not accept this unplanned conception. The lack of birth control knowledge at that time put the burden of control on the wife. She experienced feelings of shame at being pregnant during change of life. In addition, fear of retardation was great among her peers. All these factors had a strong influence on her self-image. It was not until my little sister was five years old that she came to accept this child in her heart. From that time on, my mother took over her education and became a devoted companion to her, keeping this unplanned child close to her heart and home. In her later years this daughter became her greatest consolation and pride.

Today, women having late-life or menopause pregnancies can, with good health and nutrition, give birth without fear to normal, healthy babies. Early in the pregnancy, tests of the amniotic fluid can also allay any doubts of normal development without harming the fetus. The woman has a choice.

In my experience, the soul, when perceived, manifests as a tiny, electric blue, whirling light over the belly button of the mother. As pregnancy advances, it grows in strength and size. The soul is entranced by the thought-forms created by the love relationship that exists between the couple. One could say that the soul is captured willingly. Once the soul becomes earthbound, a veil is placed between memory of the journey and manifestation. This is to encourage the soul to insist upon new experience for the purpose of soul growth.

SPIRITUAL UNION

For the spiritually oriented couple, conception is union and is a metaphor for marriage or commitment. The principle of union with God is the highest, most sacred teaching in all religious traditions. All life has within it the divine. Creating life is creating the divine and bringing it down to the earth plane. Union to the lovers is the act of seeing the divine perfection in the beloved mate. Entrancement with physical attributes causes thought-forms to impress the genetic pattern as half of the male chromosomes line up with half of the female chromosomes in twenty-three matched pairs. The qualities admired in each mate have been idealized up to the point of the physical union. In union, the glance from the eye of the beloved to the lover becomes the single-pointed concentration that true union demands. This is the beginning of both the annihilation of the limited ego and the union beyond reason or thinking. In surrender, a new state of consciousness is born. The lover completely identifies with the beloved. This is conscious conception. Couples desiring conscious conception must eradicate from mind all fear that they will lose consciousness of self. The stage of sexual desire where all fear is dissolved often happens in teenage conceptions, but the will to procreate is not conscious, nor is the dedication to the spiritual value of the act.

In India, older women have taught the young bride to understand what is expected of her, her fulfillment as a woman, and her attitude toward the male. A woman knows she has the power of the Divine Mother to lift the man into higher concepts of his self-image, into his self-realization, and into his capabilities to succeed in the world. That is the duty of the spiritual woman.

Few women today know that in mating, at the point of completion for the man, she has the mastery of breath and the power of her heart and emotional being to lift the spirit of the man into the higher centers. Instead, she often comes down to meet him and loses herself in his emotional completion. This is not the part of a spiritual mother. Rather, the spiritual mother and spiritual wife lifts the man while he does his own work. Unless she has the realization that this high point is her moment of divinity, the moment when she is the goddess, she does not realize herself. Having that realization, she can lift her man into a view of himself that he did not have previously, so that he can stand up and purify the world, with confidence to follow through with what he had, in abstract mind, conceived only in his dream states.

She can feel the emotional completion of the divinity within herself. If she is looking for that completion in her man, she is going to be disappointed. If the man is looking for it in her, he may find her very unsatisfying after the mating because she is either full of ambition to work or is unreachable and in her own world — totally separated from intercourse to intercourse. The woman may want the man to go on worshiping her as the goddess. When the sexual act is over she wonders why she is not being appreciated, why he does not see her as the most beautiful creature in the world. He does not because she herself has gotten lost in illusion. These are indications that all is not right on the inner planes; otherwise the man would feel that his mind was clear, that he could think through things and remove himself from mental and emotional traumas. If the male enters the environment of conception in the high consciousness of what procreation means, he can realize the purpose of his manhood and accept the responsibility of parenthood with joy. The maturity of mind that ensues expands his consciousness to include the family of God in a universal sense. The world he has been living in is reflected in the universe within himself. Any mating in a less than totally conscious state is only subconscious and frequently lacks bonding to the incoming soul.

Couples who have forgotten self and have been immersed in the love experience realize that their union patterns the physical vehicle that will, in 280 days or ten lunar months, house the soul at birth. True union enables the mated pair to meet soul to soul, neither possessing love, but both becoming the love principle itself; thus a child is conceived consciously.

Procreation is a physical manifestation of an act of love — a loving union, wherein the male realizes the walls of separateness between his body and that of his beloved are dissolved. "Flesh of my flesh, blood of my blood," is, for the first time, understood. On some level, they are conscious of the physical bond that takes place in the union: two germ cells, each containing half of their being, unite to become one. Uniting with the sperm, the woman's fertilized egg clings to her rich, blood-filled uterine wall. After only six days of cell division, this minute morula will burrow in and begin to distinguish its unique parts.

The couple may ponder over just when the spirit of the child entered the morula. There are diverse views, despite much scientific and metaphysical research on the subject. If one were to judge by neuromuscular action of the fetus, one would say it is at conception when the chromosomal pattern lines up, half of each parent becoming the new embryo. However, if that were true, then how can one explain many experiences that women and men recall long before conception — of the personality, the spirit, and sometimes the exact image of the physical child yet to manifest? But does the soul have to be in the body to make itself known? The spirit, when strong, impels the soul to incarnate.

Spiritual union, which we call "falling in love," is usually present in the glance long before conception. Traditionally, society blessed this experience and encouraged it to take place before the union and conception. Formalizing it with vows and religious ceremony, which we now call marriage or commitment (another rite of passage), evolved later. Conception, then, is an expression of what already exists in the love commitment. Today, commitment may be entered into in an experimental way in order to test in the fire of everyday living the ability of two people to build something positive in each other's personalities. Not all commitments lead to marriage, but all true marriages confirm the act of commitment. The couple confirms the depths of their love for their chosen ideal of womanhood or manhood through marriage.

The spiritual bond between the mating couple is forever sealed within the child at conception. The procreative act is highly sacred, as the birth is reminiscent of the divine union of God and man in the garden of Eden.

Actually, conception, pregnancy, and growth of the child can be thought of as a metaphor for courtship and marriage. Just as marriage goes through five stages, so are there five stages to conception and pregnancy that are parallel, but not synonymous with the five stages of marriage.

FIVE STAGES OF MARRIAGE

The courtship before marriage is the anticipatory dream stage that parallels the sexual anticipation before a couple makes love. Life is thrilling, every moment away from the beloved is wasted time. Only the hours spent together have meaning. The future of the relationship is "all roses" and embodies many dreams, hopes, and visions of what one could be if one would be — the dream of what one hopes for.

The first stage is followed by the honeymoon stage, where the action takes place without either mate thinking of the consequences. Each sees the other in a golden aura of perfect attributes. The glance belongs only to the beloved. Every effort is made to act, live, and be perfect in the other's eyes. Both are at their very best, trying to preserve the perfect image that they know inwardly will be recalled in memory as the ideal image.

The third stage is the awakening from the dreamlike fantasy to find that the boring routine of daily living must be faced. The letdown into the humdrum of each day allows each to fall back into the habits natural to the old, premarital self. The little quirks in human nature cause aggravation. "He's not perfect!" "She's not perfect!" How disillusioning this is. Both ask themselves, "How could I have been so fooled?" Both personalities are picked apart and observed in a new and often disillusioning light. This stage of disenchantment arrives when the necessity of working as a team is realized. The ideal must be broken if fantasy is to be destroyed. Settling for a little less than perfection must occur. When the romantic ideal that we were raised to believe through fairy tales, movies, and TV love stories is destroyed and thrown away, then true marital love on a level of peace and contentment takes over.

The fourth stage is the resignation to the best and worst in each other. Making the best of it and finding ways of walking around each other's foibles surprisingly develops strengths that balance the mate's weaknesses. A marriage has been attained at last.

Finally, the realization comes that the things that once aggravated one were really the reflections of the lacks in one's own image. A lovely plateau of peace and acceptance is reached. This whole process usually takes five years to attain or to fall apart due to the lack of willingness to build a firm foundation out of two people's individual and often opposing desires. Working through the difficulties as a team is the deepening experience.

Although the commitment makes accommodation for the process of conception and parenting, conception occurs long before the sperm unites with the egg. This is tacitly acknowledged in the expressions adults sometimes use to describe where the child was before being born: "You were a light in your daddy's eye" or "You were a thought in the back of my head."

With unplanned conceptions, although few can admit it to themselves at the time, there is a subconscious desire in one or both of the lovers for a child. This often causes the woman to take a chance that, with rational thought, she would not have dared. Many single parents have had this experience: the young woman subconsciously desires to seal the commitment and finds this feeling is not shared by the male.

Today, with women's consciousness of fertility often externalized with many types of birth control, women are sometimes unaware that they are pregnant for several months. Maureen is a single parent who explained: "I was totally unconscious about my first three pregnancies, since spiritually, I was still unawakened. Before the fourth conception, however, the father was aware of a soul hanging around whenever we were together, waiting for a commitment. I did not wish marriage and I felt the soul hesitated until I came to the point of accepting it." The unawakened parent may have no attunement to the soul's attempts at embodiment, although people using drugs in conjunction with procreating may feel like they made contact with a soul. Later they question the experience.

When conception takes place with two spiritually awakened parents, however, the presence of the incoming soul cannot be doubted. The experience of having been chosen as the parents because of the power of their love-expanded energy field is definite. It takes a great deal of presence of mind on their part to deny embodiment to that hovering soul.

FIVE STAGES OF CONCEPTION

Conception involves five stages for the mother- and father-to-be. The first stage really begins when a woman's and man's glance meet and the magnetic charge is transferred from eye to eye as the light of soul shines forth from each. Soul recognizes soul in a glance and infatuation begins. It is really in this moment that the conception of the idea of the child takes place. In such a magical moment a magnetic charge is struck from the energy field of each body and what we refer to as sexual attraction begins. This electromagnetic field is not of one body or another but is melded or incorporated from a pattern of the biological being of each; it transcends reason. An illusion is born and each sees the other in a transfigured state that we call "being in love." Reason and denial succumb as the enchantment takes over. Self-awareness is temporarily muted and another personality dominates sane reasoning. Conception that began in the mind of man transmutes in the heart of woman. The ray of the Divine Light in the glance of their eyes, which met for the first time, has kindled the flame of love.

The second stage begins when the magnetic attraction grows into a restless pulling to be in each other's presence day and night. Each creates an ideal of the other's traits — the way he walks, the way she laughs, the color of eyes, the wisp of hair, the perfume of the personality — each seems cast in perfection to the other. The perfection is so alluring that each yearns to be one with the other through mating in order to escape the unbearable separateness.

In the third stage idealization of each other's traits manifests in dream and fantasy. Awakening of the heart attracts souls anxious to become one with that vibration.

The fourth stage is the dream awakening, during the sexual consummation. The private and very secret inner self of the male must and does let go in order to reach union with the Divine Mother. The stage is set for the divine drama as hovering souls seeking embodiment interfere with the single-minded concentration of the mating couple. The lovers at first fear to speak of this to each other. But the incoming soul is not to be fended off so simply. In dreams it makes its being known to the woman and through sound it very often names itself to the male. The whole atmosphere is charged. The electromagnetic fields of male and female energy charge each other as the energy of positive and negative poles meet. Awakened and aware couples often intuitively feel the presence of souls in their dreams. Sometimes the atmosphere is felt to be charged with an unmistakable current that is made audible to the couple. Tiny lights with rotating wings or vibratory presences are sometimes seen or felt hovering over a mating made high from the procreative energy. In some cases, the whole atmosphere is charged with a heavy perfume that cannot be named. All living things take on an aura of magic. Softness of breezes never felt before and odors of perfume too delicate to come from a bottle are sensed. The elements of wind, sun, and rain are often a part of this scene.

As the years progress, each following conception is a separate and different experience from the previous one. Each soul comes with its own urgency, cyclically returning on the phases of the moon, until it is strong enough to overcome its chosen family's resistance and its own weakness or fears of grounding to this plane. In choosing its parents, the soul has been impressed from the higher planes and brings to the family qualities not yet cultivated. Each conception affects every member of the family differently. The souls that come to the mother preceding the second conception may also manifest in dreams as a strong presence or in vision as an old personality. The soul qualities of second or later children have a relationship to the first child. It will become a spiritual challenge to extend consciousness within that child, who must make room in his or her heart to accept the new sibling as a "gift from heaven" or as an "albatross around the neck." Only strong souls will be attracted to manifest in families where a first child is already well-established. Gentle souls become followers of the firstborn and observe life for many years before realizing they can take the initiative to discover their own life purpose. A third or fourth child may be called in by a firstborn child, who often informs the mother before she, herself, is aware of it.

The fifth stage is more than a physical act. It is a rite of passage in which the girl lays down her youth and rises to mature womanhood. The male passes through a similar rite of passage with the new undertaking of responsibility. The relationship between man and woman changes forever at this point.

After the conception, there is sometimes wonderment and questioning, particularly by the woman, as to just when conception began. Even if the man or woman had experienced the presence of the soul, the rational mind often steps in with doubts. A working mother confided to me, "I've always felt I missed something precious in my life by not knowing when I conceived any of my five children. I would always dream of a baby visiting me before I knew I was pregnant, but we never planned them. They just came along in their own good time."

DESECRATION OF PROCREATION

Of course, all conceptions are not divine unions. Conceptions resulting from rape, incest, or experimentation with the lower self-gratifying centers result in prolonged and intense emotional and mental suffering. The inevitable battle between the lower and higher selves detains the fulfillment of womanhood and discourages acceptance of the incoming soul. When procreation deteriorates into recreation, the sacredness of the act is desecrated, the divine sinks to the mundane and the woman or man is stopped in his/her cycle of developmental maturation. The whole purpose of life is denied. Spiritual and psychological counseling should be sought within the first weeks of such pregnancies.

In the case of rape, when the thought-forms in procreation are negative and nonexistent, and only fear and escape are in the mind of the woman, all systems of the body give the alarm and trauma ensues. Society has acknowledged that conception resulting from rape is no spiritual union, which is why it has always been legal to abort in such cases.

In ancient societies, the taboos of the clan or tribe protected the immature from desecrating the procreative act. In our society, where mores are collapsing at a rapid rate, only the reverence for life and personal relationships will assure immortality of the race and will revitalize the society.

1. Neumann, Erich. *The Great Mother — An Analysis of the Archetype.* Princeton: Princeton University Press, 1974.

2. "Hypnotized children recall birth experiences — mother's memories verified." *BrainMind Bulletin.* Vol. 6, No. 4, 26 January 1981, p. 1.

3. Veeneklass. *Physicians' Bulletin.* Vol. 24, 15 January 1959.

4. Taylor and Madison, *Journal of Obstetrics and Gynecology,* Vol. 73, No. 5, October 1966, pp. 142–146.

5. Heath, Robert, M.D. Chairman, Department of Psychiatry and Neurology, Tulane Medical Center, New Orleans, Louisiana.

6. Khan, Hazrat Inayat. *The Soul Whence and Whither.* New Lebanon, N.Y.: Sufi Order Publications, 1977, p. 122.

7. Ibid., p. 105.

CHAPTER TWO

Planned Conception

Committed couples, from the day of conception onward, tend to reevaluate their own sex roles. Not age but readiness determines progress in this task. The woman first builds a normal and well-balanced physical housing for the spirit of the child to occupy at birth. Rest, relaxation, and good nutrition are a very real part of this preparation. She then may create beauty, harmony, and a loving vibration by tuning herself to all that reflects the Divine Light in flowers, art, and literature. A committed man will sustain the emotional stability of the mother by means of his concentration, mental support, and his total awareness of the new and emerging family environment. This includes building a nest within a suitable environment to impress the incoming soul with the societal value system as well as his own state of consciousness. A positive environment is one in which love and harmony permeate; in which order, cleanliness, and light produce equanimity in the human spirit. Constant moving of the nest has an adverse effect upon the stages of labor, so moves should be made early.

Mature adults accept conception as fulfillment of their human purpose and part of the soul's goal. On the physical level, both men and women planning for conception may take this opportunity to cleanse themselves of toxins, attend to diet, and discontinue any drug use or smoking or drinking habits. Balance between work and play as well as activity and repose eliminates stress buildup. Both should also be aware of their own and their mate's ancestry. The cells that are passed on to the fetus are already patterned and actively impressing the reproductive system.

Many women are quite unaware of their cyclic rhythms and fertile times, making pregnancy a mysterious unknown. The inner urge to conceive intrudes upon the old mind-set and new emotions surface. There is great value in a woman's having control of when she has her children. Making that choice makes pregnancy a joy. It takes spiritual self-discipline. A woman who learns her natural ovulation cycle makes conscious an important part of her being, enabling her to go with the positive and negative mood changes. Instead of pregnancy happening to her, conscious pregnancy or birth control should be totally her choice. Readiness for motherhood is a very individual experience; there is no universal right time in life's transitions, but rather "my right time."

For the woman who wants to plan her conception, knowledge of her fertile times is a necessity. Many well-recommended books cover natural birth control methods that utilize cervical mucus observation and basal body temperature in combination with rhythm.[1] Using a combination of such methods gives a woman real understanding and consciousness of her body. Lunaception is one method by which a woman may attain knowledge of her fertile time by means of light control and body temperature.[2] It appeals to those who practice light work at the new moon.

There are also scientific methods of selecting the gender of the child. The acidity or alkalinity of the vagina favors a boy or girl.[3] The Astrological Birth Control Centre for Planned Parenthood in Czechoslovakia claims that a woman is most fertile when the angle of the sun and moon match the time of the woman's own birth. This method has been successful 97.7 percent of the time. These studies also indicate that the moon affects the womb's alkaline-acid balance, which determines the gender of sperm that reaches and fertilizes the egg. Research shows some success in choosing the gender.[4]

The potential father, aware of the condition of his physical body, may want to consider the gifts of his seed and his family inheritance. Research may convince him to quit bad habits, such as smoking tobacco or marijuana, taking drugs, or drinking alcohol. Children who are raised in homes where one of the parents smokes are adversely affected by the smoke fumes, even when they are not themselves smokers.[5] The spiritually awakened male sees fatherhood as the fulfillment of his innermost desire for immortality.

Planned pregnancy can cultivate certain mental attitudes in the couple. Renunciation of the lower self in the making of a child dominates the love relationship. Conception at its best is attained through minds that are free of unhealthy attitudes that may remain from early childhood learning about sex; attitudes unknowingly inherited from our parents.

While keeping in mind their own attitudes toward sex, the couple must realize that they will also be forming their children's attitudes. Many old patterns surface at this time. Our parents' attitudes toward excretion and body awareness and whether we were shown pleasure and praise rather than displeasure has affected our own attitudes. Signs of mucous secretion in girl babies and erections in boy babies should be greeted casually and with signs of pleasure, so that children of both sexes may develop pride in their sexuality. Reactions of squeamishness or displeasure may inhibit later mating instincts.

It is convincing to consider other cultures' sociosexual mores to broaden our views and free ourselves of preconceived notions about our own sexuality. Where skin contact through sleeping in the same bed with brothers and sisters in childhood was the prevalent lifestyle, as with the Amish in Pennsylvania and the Manus in New Guinea, masturbation and early pregnancies do not, as a rule, exist. The need for skin contact, massage, and body security is something modern societies have lost sight of in the civilization process, thus omitting an important aspect of natural acceptance of the body. Patting, hugging, and play build emotionally secure adults who conceive in full awareness.

Conscious conception demands that men and women acknowledge their readiness for responsibility. For the woman, this means preparing herself to devote the first two-and-a-half years to childcare in order to lay the groundwork for an emotionally healthy, whole child. Of course, if the parents merely open up to the incoming soul, tuning in to the fetus, they will find that preparation for each following stage of pregnancy will come naturally. Pregnancy and lactation hormones prepare the woman for the nesting just as false menstrual cramps and Braxton-Hicks contractions prepare her for waking up several times a night without feeling loss of sleep the next day.

SPIRITUAL ASPECTS OF CONCEPTION

The spiritual aspects of conception determine the kind of caretaker the mother will be. The angelic soul manifests on this plane not only to be guided and nurtured, but also because it has things to teach and gifts to give. From conception forward, it must always be remembered that the child is not possessed by the parents, but is only a temporary visitor. What follows is a conception meditation — a concentration inviting the soul into the couple's life. Begin with the invocation to the angels of love:

> O angels of love, Theliel, Rahmeil, Raphael, Donquel, Liwet, and Anael, guide the soul who has chosen my womb to build the temple of God that it will occupy on earth. O blessed angels, created by the breath of God, send a soul to me/us who embodies the most blessed of Thy Divine Attributes, _____ [name the qualities you desire]. Through the light of Lailah, angel of conception, grant my heart's desire and make me a worthy guardian to this incoming soul. Amen.

The couple may find that a meditation on the star of Bethlehem is appropriate. Individually inspired symbols may be drawn, painted, or sewn and hung in the bedroom. For a contemplation, Sufi Order West suggests using the following symbol:

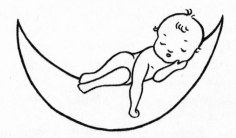

Social and moral aspects of conception also need to be looked at. A few close friendships with other couples, preferably with those who are planning their own child, are great assets. Maintaining or reviving family ties can also be a great support. It is helpful to take a critical look at current career and educational goals as well as financial management after birth. The current lifestyle will also have to be reevaluated by both parents. When communication is kept open, each is more capable of supporting the other. Open communication also encourages expression of innermost feelings of misunderstanding that make for extended stages of labor in birthing. Be totally honest with each other where fears or reservations are concerned. It is quite normal to have ambivalent feelings in the first six weeks.

ENVIRONMENTAL QUALITY

The quality of the environment is an increasingly important factor in holistic living. In large metropolitan areas where the air, water, soil, and vegetation are likely to be polluted to varying degrees, considering a move to a more healthy living environment is advisable. The proliferation of nuclear power plants is an infectious social blight not to be overlooked. If the couple is living near a nuclear reactor, it would be wise to leave the area. The government may have been negligent in not publicizing the tragedies that occurred and are still occurring since the March 1979 Three Mile Island nuclear power plant disaster. Only foreign newspapers and journals seem to carry an honest representation of what has happened there. The number of reported infant deaths rose 92 percent during the three to four months following the disaster in the areas within the path of the radioactive plume of gases. Radioactive iodine was responsible for the infant deaths and miscarriages, not only of human babies, but of livestock as well.[6] Wisdom precludes any choice of living near such areas.

The natural environment in which a couple plans to conceive a child is a very present health consideration whenever the waters are polluted with pesticides, herbicides, nitrates, sewage, artificial fertilizers, and other toxic chemicals that also plague the earth. The air is full of industrial carcinogens, lead, carbon monoxide, and other toxic substances. However, it is likely that those in high states of consciousness will be able to transmute and survive in our polluted world. Excessive worry, however, over the ruining of the planet leads to stress and health problems and interferes with the perception of the divine purpose of conception.

The home environment, however, is within the control of the couple, who should strive to build a secure, healthy, reflective, and loving space for the incoming soul. It is particularly the woman's spiritual purpose to maintain the subtle atmosphere in the home, inviting only those persons whom she intuitively feels will aid in building her nest and in tuning the vibration to a higher degree of refinement than ever before.

INABILITY TO CONCEIVE

For the couple who seems unable to have children, planning a family involves several options: artificial insemination (which accounts for several thousand births per year in the United States), hormones, surgery, or adoption. The latter is often the remedy for stressed, nervous couples who have no physical explanation for their lack of conception. Relaxation and enjoyment of the adopted baby is often followed by a surprise conception of their own child. Spiritually speaking, these people have realized only the mental part of conception — they have probably doubted their own manhood and womanhood and have worried themselves into states of further self-doubt. Caring for and playing with other people's children often aids the woman in relaxing and gaining confidence in nurturing. The male who can gain confidence in his manhood in a sport, hobby, or other self-confidence-inspiring activity may let down blocks in his psyche, thus attaining a new approach to the act of love. He then may become a natural father if all tests show no physical cause for sterility.

MISCARRIAGE AND INFANT DEATH

After conception, sometimes the soul is not strong enough to manifest on our plane and must return to its djinn world or astral plane to gain further strengthening. Perhaps the magnetism of one or both lovers is not strong enough to give power for breathing rhythmically. This accounts for many miscarriages and infant deaths. It seems there are many souls trying to reembody that are not sufficiently strengthened before they return, perhaps because of trauma and shortened life span due to starvation, war, or migration. Especially after sudden death, which enhances the desire to come back, souls will often immediately try to return and continue the former life in another body. And if there is not a strong enough impulse, the fetus cannot live. The impulse on that fetus cannot hold; then the soul cannot embody. But it will return until the energy field produced by the love relationship of the individual mother is such that embodiment is assured, always in the right time and place.

In cases of repeated or late miscarriage, the mourning process is very real for the couple. There is an intensity of loss that comes after miscarriage, when it is seemingly impossible for that mother to release the infant that has been miscarried. The intensity and duration of the mourning period will vary according to how much she associated with that soul. Ways of associating or connecting with the fetus include putting the hand on the abdomen and feeling the presence of the entity, tuning in to it, and visually and mentally sending it love and encouragement. This concentration may even take the form of repulsion if she was still fighting it or had not made up her mind. When a successive pregnancy follows a miscarriage too closely, the mother often carries the mourning process over to the new fetus; it is difficult to separate them. Communicating grief to friends, mates, or support groups eases and hastens the mourning period.

Mourning for a fetus or an infant goes through stages, and is not limited to the mother; fathers also may experience mourning. One man clung to his fetus son's image for years because a mourning ritual had been avoided, until at last he was able to let it go.

During the first stage the parents cannot mentally accept what has happened. They often exclaim, "I can't accept it; I can't realize it; it has happened, yet I can't believe it." The second stage is the feeling of complete shock and helplessness. They cannot reason about it and do not know what to do or how they are going to adjust or live with the tragedy. The third stage is substitution, when some family member or friend steps in and shares the grief. In the days when there were larger nuclear families, with relatives who were also having babies, the mother could compensate her loss with caring for another infant. It tended to make the mourning process easier and to end it faster. When this substitution process does not happen, the period of grief can go on for a long time. Today, it is normally a two-year period.

The last stage of mourning is relinquishment. The couple must be willing to send the soul back so that it can get more strength to return, or must be able to relinquish the soul entirely to another plane, without clinging. The hardest thing in the world is to let go, especially of a dream or an emotional bond. To relinquish, the father and mother may place the lost child with a guardian angel, or hold the child's image in their memory, recalling the child's birthday or beauty, which in time

becomes a part of their minds and hearts. This is a spiritual relinquishing. Particularly for the mother, the support and understanding of her mate will enable her to accept the death and
relinquish that child. Burying the remains and planting a tree
helps.

When the parents have given themselves time to go through
the mourning stages, sharing their grief, the wounds will heal
faster. If disrupted because of resistance to relinquishment, the
mourning process takes a longer time — as much as ten years,
according to investigations by psychologists. Some women hold
onto their loss, thereby preventing themselves from being fulfilled in another pregnancy or in service. This type of woman
does not substitute her loss with other people's infants or try to
serve humanity with work in schools or with children's hospitals, but just keeps clinging to the sorrow, often in silence.
There is no greater cure than going outside of one's own group
to serve others. Nurturing another infant and involvement with
infant and childcare programs works toward a completion and
true release from guilt and self-recrimination of any kind.

When a couple is able to speak to other parents about grief
feelings, the pain eases. It is often difficult to discuss these
feelings in our society, where shyness and respect for grief, or
total ignorance about death, cover the need for communication
of the stages of grief. In cases of stillbirth, particularly, it is important for the parents to relinquish the soul; otherwise the experience could interfere with bonding in the next pregnancy.
For the mother, positive goals of rebuilding her body through
wise nutrition and of occupying her time in some gratifying social service while preparing positively for a second pregnancy
lessen the pain and promote faith in the future.

ABORTION

Unplanned pregnancies may challenge the woman in a
quite different way. The decision to carry or abort should ideally be made by both the pregnant woman and the father of the
child. Many women feel that it is their right to accept or reject

motherhood totally on their own. Today, when there is free choice, a woman tends to delay and ponder until the third month to come to terms with her pregnant condition. Forty or fifty years ago, women had to make this decision early or not consider it at all. The third month is the period when the fetus has made up its mind, its development is progressing rapidly but, due to her lack of acceptance, it is not having the nurturing or magnetizing that it should have. She very seldom tells her husband or lover about it until she has made up her own mind, or she may not tell him at all, if he is not free of another relationship.

The awakened father is aware of the pregnancy and helps to nurture the incoming soul by adding his magnetism — in massaging the mother's back, in the meeting of skin and of hands, and in the exchange of energies in intercourse. The cupping of the hands over the shoulder blades (which Inayat Khan says are reminders of our angel wings — the wings of light) brings the oneness of the Light Being within the spheres of light to the couple's perception. It can be considered the esoteric part of our coming together. So little of this unifying is done consciously or is even understood by women. Meanwhile, conflict between her heart and mind and peers' opinions carries the woman's thoughts around in circles, causing her further emotional turmoil and prolonging decision making. Feelings of inadequacy and inability to face motherhood often lead to confusion and abrupt decisions to terminate the pregnancy.

In some cases, modern abortion methods fail to terminate the pregnancy and the mother has to go back to have it completed. The fetus just does not want to let go. This attachment by the fetus may be caused by a father who, although he hesitates to influence her, does not want the woman to make the decision against her deepest emotional desire and deeper love nature. She may have a very difficult time accepting the abortion by reason alone. If she cannot accept it, it will affect her emotional body. Once this occurs, she is likely to be unable to reason about it at all. When a woman is emotionally upset she is likely to be mentally unreasonable — a difficult situation for the thinking male to contend with. The stronger the rejection in the mother's mental and emotional bodies, the stronger the new soul will show itself to be. This trauma can have a detrimental effect on the woman because when she is uptight, it affects the uterus or other organs. When a man is uptight, it usually begins in his head; mentally he just tightens up, cannot think, gets angry with himself, impatient with his household, and his friendships are strained.

Previous abortions or miscarriages that left the mother feeling unloved or unsupported can precipitate fear for her health or for the survival of the new infant and retard the early bonding during pregnancy. Often abortions result in a secondary crisis that may continue for years, affecting inner feelings of self-worth, causing distrust of males, and often resulting in many broken relationships and the inability of the woman to practice birth control. Psychic disturbance can grow out of the mate's rejection of the responsibility of fatherhood, which can be misinterpreted by the woman as her being unworthy of carrying his baby. She may blame herself for ruining a relationship that was happy prior to the conception. Unfounded fears of hereditary weakness in her family may haunt her. The right-to-life movement has given a new view of easy abortion and its consequences. Immature men, unwilling to accept adult responsibility, influence insecure women to abort. Guidance and objective counseling should be sought early.

Emotional and mental turmoil may not be the only causes for considering abortion. For every couple who faces genetic disease it must be an individual decision. "If you don't know the soul of the child the decision to abort will be easier, but if you know and have met that being, you simply could not do it," Pir Vilayat Khan, head of the Sufi Order of the West, has said.

The spiritually awakened woman who has been forced by circumstances or an act of God to accept abortion as a solution, must come to terms with her own conscience. If the thought is present that abortion is the murder of a part of herself, then she cannot and should not abort. But if the woman sees the fetus as only the housing or accommodation for the soul, with birth as the "housewarming," then abortion can be an acceptable choice. Even when one sees the physical apparatus only as the housing for the soul of the child, it is a desecration to destroy it before the tenant can move in. Destruction by will and intent calls for some kind of reparation to the soul who suffered the trauma of abortion, as well as to the psyche of the one responsible for that decision. By making a conscious effort to contact the rejected soul and by explaining and confessing her sorrow (which she also shares with others), the woman will be able to heal the scar for them both. She may also perform acts of good intent to other souls entering this plane. Only through acts that consciously restore life to lower kingdoms and by sending thought-forms of explanation to the rejected soul can the guilt be dissolved.

1. Nofziger. *A Cooperative Method of Birth Control.* 2d ed., revised, Summertown, Tenn.: Book Publishing Co., 1978.

2. Lacey, Louise. *Lunaception — A Feminine Odyssey into Fertility and Contraception.* New York: Warner Books, 1974.

3. Rodale, J.I. *Nutrition, Health and Pregnancy.* New York: Pyramid Books, 1968, pp. 78–80.

4. Rorvik, David, and Landrum Shettles. *Your Baby's Sex — Now You Can Choose.* New York: Bantam Books, 1970, pp. 37–40.

5. Ostrander and Shroeder. Astrological Birth Control Centre, Czechoslovakia; Jonas, Eugen, *Behind the Iron Curtain.*

6. Fawlick, Thomas. "The Silent Toll," *Harrowsmith Magazine.* Ontario, Canada, 1980, pp. 33–49.

CHAPTER THREE

Unplanned Conception

A majority of the conceptions in the United States are unplanned. In our complex and rapidly changing society, accepting the unplanned conception does not only occur within traditional committed or nurturing relationships that are specifically designed for raising children. Many girls in their early teens as well as older, experienced women are conceiving without wishing to. With husbands or without; with committed male friends or in communities; with marriage plans or freelance, it still happens endlessly in the eighties. For these women, the ability to accept the changes that conception brings are determined by many diverse factors. The context surrounding unplanned conception has much to do with attitudes toward parenting, either negatively or positively patterned by upbringing.

There is a growing trend in our society for teenaged girls to become single mothers. In a culture where there are many well-publicized birth control clinics and available counseling, it is sometimes difficult for adults to understand why this is happening. One mother in ten is pregnant before the age of eighteen, and ten-, eleven-, and twelve-year-old girls are getting pregnancy tests.[1] The teenaged girl accepts the role of recreation partner and then finds that the joy of procreation is not shared. The consequent painful confrontation with parents, interrupted social life, lowered self-esteem, and increased worry take over her personality. For the modern teenage girl, this can be a debilitating experience.

Governed and nurtured by a strong peer group morality,

she is easily led into believing that intercourse feels good and that it assures being loved and wanted. However, after conception, the relationship with her lover can often end in rejection, perhaps after several years of faithfulness, leaving a deep scar on the psyche of the young woman. Seldom is any contraceptive used in the first months, as young girls often feel that they cannot become pregnant. Parenthood and its hazards begin to loom large with a rude awakening to the fact that the father of her child does not choose to share responsibility for parenting it. Walking away from the teenaged mother is no longer frowned upon in his peer group. Today, society has been forced to accept the teenage mother and child because of their prevalence. Welfare programs subsidize her and she has found a way to leave her parents' home and to live her own life in her own way.

During the 1980s, when the mate rejects the responsibility of fatherhood, an increasing number of young women are choosing single parenthood rather than abortion or adoption. This is possible, to a large extent, because social services, single parent associations, and society aid the single parent in her commitment to mothering her own child. The road is not an easy one, however, for the single parent.

Since the sixties, single parents have become a substantial segment of the population. In the eighties, "one-third of all families with children are headed by a single parent. Furthermore, statistics project that half of all children born in 1980 will spend part of their childhood years in a home with only one parent."[2] In view of this large group, the following section, regarding reactions of various people to their conceiving a child, is divided into married or committed-relationship parents and single parents.

CONCEPTION TESTS COUPLES AND COMMUNITIES

The following accounts concern parents who are married or in committed relationships. Since there are many challenges to meet and tests to pass en route to parenthood, particularly for the woman who becomes pregnant and marries soon after, the rite is a major transition in life. At the very least, it demands nurturing and housekeeping, and sometimes it calls for aid in financially supporting the home. Such young relationships place stress on the personal growth and self-esteem of the woman. At the same time, the man committed to accepting fatherhood as a mature adult gains both spiritually and mentally.

Lisa and Tom, both in their mid-twenties, had waited to have a baby until they had completed their vocational training. They had observed and talked with friends who had already started their families. They located a community and built their own nest with the help of their friends. They were well-read on the subject and felt that their relationship had evolved to a stable place and that they had developed real values for parenting. Their conception was planned for a general "right time."

Tom had deeply rooted protective instincts toward all children. He wanted to be a very real part of the pregnant-couple experience. As soon as he finished building his home, Tom furnished the room in which he planned to conceive his child. After the birth, I visited the baby and Lisa told me, wistfully, in a moment alone, "I really never felt I'd conceived this baby until I felt it kick. Tom had waited so long that he had a mental image all ready. When our baby was born, Tom cried out, 'He's just like I saw him the night we conceived him!'" Tom was that rare pioneer American father who delivered his own baby, washed and dressed him, and bonded himself to his son completely. Lisa nursed him and the rest of the time Tom did everything necessary, working a broken shift to adjust to the baby's nurturing. I consoled her, "Why don't you surprise him next time?" Not all women may be nurturing types, but some men certainly are.

In communities where group marriage is practiced, everyone in the community takes responsibility for the child's support and caretaking. Where the woman has conceived without knowledge of her fertile times, some interesting relationships develop. One such lady came to me for counseling regarding her nine-year-old daughter's fathering problems.

> All of the three men who might have been responsible for Dharma's conception have continued to remain close with us. All of the men have been called "uncle" by my daughter, but now the physical resemblance between one of them and my daughter is unmistakable to the group. (The man I am presently married to is not her father.) Dharma has a special relationship with her blood father, although he recently left the group to marry and now has a child by that marriage. I don't know whether to tell her the truth now or let her believe that my present mate is her father."

David and Roslyn were a couple who had grown children and Roslyn was going through menopause when she became pregnant without knowing it. Since they had experienced one stillbirth caused by a genetic disease, Roslyn became hysterical with worry.

David sought genetic counseling at once to find out what the risk of recurrence would be. Both of them recalled the shock, bewilderment, and fear (and in David's case, the anger) they had experienced at the time of the stillbirth. Both had vowed never to have another child. After all, they were lucky to have had two normal boys. How could they take a chance on that extra chromosome or that mutant gene? This traumatic event demanded immediate attention.

Roslyn needed supportive counseling while David demanded expert genetic counseling. Since the diagnosis was not clear, they returned to their own physician, who knew the family well. The chromosomal disease called "Klinefelter's syndrome" was explained to them as the presence of an extra chromosome that has a low but definite risk of recurrence. Prenatal monitoring was available to them. Roslyn sought spiritual counseling and David went along with it, but it was psychological counseling that made up his mind. He summed it up like this:

We came home exhausted from the third session with different doctors. Vague help was offered by the psychologist, who felt that time was needed to work with us separately, since Roslyn was in such mental and emotional turmoil. We wanted a quick answer and felt we were just getting the runaround. The minister had told us to go home and pray for an answer to our problem and then to meditate. Roslyn wanted to try it. In that first desperate attempt we did not expect much, but both of us experienced the presence of the child's spirit. If there was ever a mental conception, we both felt we experienced it at this time of crisis. Roslyn decided to go through with the pregnancy, with my full backup. Our little girl was born normal and healthy and has been the greatest joy to us both. I'm glad we took the risk.

Naomi was twelve years old when she started her sex life. At school, she and her peers were exposed to sex education classes that included lessons in contraception. When asked if she had knowledge of the chances she took, Naomi answered:

Oh yes, I heard the lectures but I guess I just wasn't ready to listen. I never believed that it could happen to me. Other girls told me that intercourse felt good, that my parents knew this and that only a 'dork' would pass up the good times one could have on weekends. Jim gave me plenty of attention until I told him I was pregnant. That he couldn't take, so he ran away. I remembered the love we had and decided to have my baby and support it myself. It was a good excuse to get away from home anyhow. My divorced mother had her own life to live, as she let me know.

Perhaps such experiences as Naomi's suggest that subconsciously the girl wants to be pregnant. Assisted by friends, welfare agencies, state education, and job training programs, many teenaged girls manage to succeed in mothering, overcoming the constant struggle that is the single parent's lot. The fortunate ones may meet child-oriented young men who take over the father-image role to their children, for the child needs both male and female models to learn from. At daycare centers, it is obvious when children are without a father and are starved for male energy, for they cling to their male caretaker (if fortunate enough to have such a father image), and emulate him. Very often, the single mother lives with other women in similar circumstances and tries to continue her education or job training. Or perhaps, if it was religious or moral standards that influenced the girl to continue the pregnancy, she seeks out community living for support.

SEX EDUCATION OF YOUTHS

Human reproduction classes are taught too late in our classrooms or at developmental ages when the students are simply not interested. We should teach human reproduction to children of junior-high-school age, when sexual interest begins. The increase in young teenage pregnancies that began in the late 1970s will not decrease until we bridge the mental gap between the sex act and conception. Unless counselors are allowed to encourage parents to provide such teaching, parents may continue to invite early pregnancies through lack of or poor communication about sexuality.

We must first teach the purpose of life so that youths can attain reverence for giving life. Nonsexual outlets must be given so that adulthood may be attained with some awareness of life's purpose. Self-control must be introduced in infancy and rewarded consistently by caretakers in the early years. Rites of passage, such as the Bar Mitzvah and Bat Mitzvah in Judaism, are valuable experiences that can introduce children to valuable nonsexual aspects of becoming adults.

Even when the mature young woman in her twenties or early thirties conceives without consciously planning for it, the magic of the relationship may be dissolved by the man's inability to face the mature responsibilities that fathering demands. The male who conceives a child without commitment to the female partner stops his spiritual advancement for lack of responsibility.

SINGLE-PARENTHOOD DECISIONS

There is always trauma and confusion surrounding single conception experiences during the first ninety days. This is not surprising in a society that has evolved in little more than two hundred years, where there is little tradition to look toward for stability. This bewilderment over conception is particularly present in the climate of today's vacillating sexual roles. Society offers numerous conflicting roles to model, but many are not in keeping with patterning children in the first two years of life.

If the woman has been successful and competent in her work and is a creative, independent person, she will probably take pride in her single parenthood, associating with women's groups and welfare agencies that will give her backup during her pregnancy. The teenager may use the conception of her baby as an excuse to get away from home and authority. The awakened woman in her late twenties or thirties, disillusioned by a partner unwilling to accept fatherhood, will take the experience as her God-given right and courageously do it alone. She may have to fight to retain her job during pregnancy, and appeal to women's rights organizations for support. Her dilemma will be whether to keep any contact with the man or to make a complete break, supported only by trusted friends.

Single women react quite differently to pregnancy. Serena, a woman in her mid-twenties who lived in a spiritual community with her partner, also faced the dilemma of aborting or sacrificing the happy sexual relationship of five years because the man she believed loved her could not face fatherhood. Opting for single parenthood, she left the community and, assisted by her friends, welfare, and her own income from work in another branch of the community, allowed the father visitation rights in the hope that the fathering instinct would develop in him through association with the child. It took seven years for this to happen and by then, Serena had outgrown the need for the relationship.

Miriam, a thirty-year-old businesswoman found herself in a similar position. "I did not find out that he was a married man until I became pregnant. Since he did not intend to divorce his wife and I did not intend to abort a soul that was very real to me at conception, it became clear that, regardless of the opinions of our business associates, I intended to have my child and to continue my career." She went to court, sought complete custody of her child, and accepted no financial aid from the father. She won her case. Conception developed a power and determination in Miriam that manifested under pressure, to her own surprise. This same power and determination aids many women on the difficult path of single parenthood.

1. Smith, Peggy B., and David M. Mumford, eds. *Adolescent Pregnancy: Perspective for the Health Professional.* Boston: G.K. Hall, 1980.

2. "White House Conference on Families," *Baby Talk*, Vol. 45, No. 8, August 1980, p. 9.

CHAPTER FOUR

Pregnancy

In the first phase of pregnancy the mixed receptivity between the earthly and heavenly kingdoms causes mixed emotions in the mother-to-be. The spiritual life of the new mother will change as the reality of the commitment to have her child is accepted. The woman often desires to spend her silent times increasingly alone in nature. Every mother learns in time to pray. As the full implication of being the first spiritual guide seeps in she often finds that entering into a life of contemplation and prayer paves the way to the relinquishment of self-love. To love is to give unstintingly of herself. Her recent mating confirms this realization. In the planting of the seed, the love is consummated, as the couple asks nothing other than to unconditionally give to each other of themselves. As self-love and love for her mate and their child are integrated into one emotion, the confusion phase melts away. A feeling of joyous fulfillment and adventure in getting to know the new soul takes place.

The relinquishment of her old pattern of life for a new attunement with the entering soul and growing fetus demands that she come to terms with herself. For the woman, giving of self may be followed by unforeseeable, unpredictable consequences, such as changing goals, careers, friendships, and commitments.

At first she may not feel mature enough to face motherhood or the loss of her future, her figure, or sex appeal. After awhile, however, the protective instinct grows and it becomes her desire to discipline herself for nine months in order to create out of her physical, spiritual, emotional, and mental fiber the most perfect vehicle possible to harbor the entering soul.

PSYCHOSPIRITUAL ADJUSTMENT FOR THE EXPECTANT MOTHER

The pregnant woman now starts to think of two beings: herself and the fetus within her womb. Looking forward to pregnancy as an adventure enables her to enjoy the many fetal changes that will affect her body, heart, and soul. She will learn an entirely new communication, where listening begins from within and registers on the eardrum. The months ahead will be full of surprises that cannot be foreseen, since each pregnancy is different. No two are alike in development of the inner self that accompanies fetal development, but every woman going through this inner change must expand her consciousness. This renunciation of her old self-image will disturb her most in the first weeks. Accepting the new responsibility is at first frightening.

This anxiety comes about during pregnancy, when subconscious fears become a force in reorganizing old goals and objectives. Separating the new image of physical self from inner self is the first challenge. Adjusting the psyche and personality to the temperament of the new entity calls for changes in attitude. Faith in the purpose of her life and the positive outcome of her commitment to mothering must be reinforced by those around her. Particularly today, parenting demands strength and resourcefulness to meet the deterioration of the old society and the faltering of the economy. Talking out fears with one's mate, a close friend, or the birthing coach or midwife can help clear the psyche for a joyous emergence into the new role of first guide to the child.

Perhaps in pondering women throughout the ages who bore and raised children or in reading about the lives of pioneer women in America who, alone in a new land, found the courage to birth and care for their babies, the newly pregnant mother may ask, "How did they do it? What was the secret of their faith and belief in themselves as mothers?" She may then remind herself that there is an ancient rhythm that brought her own mother and grandmother safely into the world. That rhythm, when she masters her breath, will give secure faith in her own child's birth and her ability to be master of herself.

The mother-to-be frequently finds herself having lengthy conversations with herself. "I'm going to be a mother, but am I ready? Will I be the kind of mother I want to be? I'm not finished working through the psychological relationship with my own parents; how will I handle being the parent of this child? I don't want this child to go through a childhood like I had! What if I drop the baby?" Such inner dialogue is a part of the natural progression that a woman goes through as soon as she accepts her pregnancy. When doubting her ability to mother, she can daily give herself positive reinforcement by saying aloud, "I am a capable, understanding, and loving person. I will be a good mother." Keeping this printed phrase in her room can impress and remind the mother-to-be to have faith and all will be well. The woman often becomes aware that the quality of her own heart is the best reinforcement and guarantee for being courageous in childbirth and strong in mothering. The quality of mothering is, after all, learned through the experience of dealing with one's own infant.

When the pregnant woman can work up from her subconscious mind her deepest anxieties, which she interprets as inadequacies to face the challenge of motherhood, she is better able to cope with the nurturing process after her baby is born. As the mind settles into peaceful thoughts and the heart adjusts to its growing intuitive powers, she may gradually resolve to accept any kind of infant that she may bear. A communion between her own moods and her baby's movements subtly makes for a new type of communication.

Since her attitudes and anticipation establish the first intrauterine relationship, she may want to build up her moral codes, courage, and self-confidence during this period. Building into her new code of ethics the mother ideal she aspires to requires putting the developing child, as a negative plate, before her mind's eye. Then she can ask herself, "What impress do I want to give my child? How can I give to this child the freedom to be a joyous and unique being, yet teach it self-control over the vicissitudes of life?" To accomplish this, her values and understanding must expand. Direct and honest communication, perhaps lacking in her own childhood, can provide the vehicle for making the ideal impress. She often resolves to develop this quality of expressive self-understanding in herself and to encourage it within her child. She may realize there is more she can do to fully communicate with her mate and may begin to work more earnestly than ever for effective communication. Making these resolutions beforehand, when love and expectations are high, is easier than after the birth, when new routines occupy the mind.

The new mother usually begins to mentally sift her personal experience and to observe other mothers. Gradually, and sometimes with vehement outbursts of realization, she may search her inner self for a new value system; one from which worthy nurturing ideals emerge. From the well of memory she can abstract the lessons learned from her own early childhood and determine the goals to pursue with her own infant.

Through searching, a new vision can be miraculously given to her. Suddenly she finds herself captivated by babies and young mothers, children with their baby-sitters, and fathers with their families. The streets seem to be crowded with pregnant women and children. This new focus marks the beginning of the mothering attribute of falling totally in love with all children. She may discover within the secret reservoir of her heart an unknown and unmeasured supply of intuition, knowledge, and love that she can tap; a resource which reassures her that she will be a good mother.

She may mentally evaluate and carefully monitor what she allows herself to focus on, finding in her heart a new sensitivity when listening to and perceiving her world. The more she clarifies her mental outlook, the more positive will be her attitudes and feelings about the role of motherhood and the smoother will be the transitions after birth into caretaker and nurturer. If she has not had younger brothers and sisters to nurture, involving herself in the care of friends' or relatives' children can build her confidence and sensitivity to an infant, alleviating the doubts and fears of her own abilities to care for her infant. Involving the father-to-be in this preparatory caretaking and in reading birthing literature is a wise way to provide a forum for evolving parenting ideals and to get the man accustomed to the vibration of the little one.

Observing how other parents handle their children in parks and public places can give both expectant parents a fuller understanding of alternatives in child guidance than reading a half dozen books on the subject. Observing the way parents of other cultures nurture their young can give particular depth and meaning to their own enculturation, as can reading widely about the customs and beliefs of other racial and ethnic groups. Through these observations further development of parenting goals are attained.

Learning about the customs and beliefs of the father's heritage (as well as understanding the mother's more fully) and exposing themselves to the father's family's views can give further meaning to the goals and ideals for raising their infant, promoting mutual understanding as they grow together. Each must attune to the values held dear by the other. Understanding the heritage of each is important for it awakens the couple to strengths as well as weaknesses of both families. Striving toward mutual attunement will help the couple to agree on their parenting goals at an early and propitious time.

As the physical body changes, so the desires of the expectant mother also change. There is a natural inclination to exercise as the skin stretches. The demand for a stable nest, protection, and peace of mind is also a natural result of the changing maternal self. The looks she gets from store clerks, neighbors, and friends, as they perceive her changing profile, affect her emotional body in a positive way. Everybody loves the glow of a pregnant woman. She is special even to strangers. Her developing intuitive receptivity to the soul of the child enables her to feel secretive or proud, to cover her growing tummy or stride forth, melon-like and radiant. Her culture and the early impress from her mother will determine how concealing or revealing her particular cloak of pregnancy will manifest in public.

Beginning with illustrations in embryology texts, the pregnant woman now visually studies with personal interest the growth of the fetus within her womb. She begins to realize that by taking the vision of the fetus developing within her body as a concentration, she can participate consciously in its growth and perfection. Protecting the fetus in those first twenty weeks, when it is so vulnerable, demands a new look at her own health regime. The white knight within her mate now emerges to become a protector. Taking all precautions, avoiding all risks, she begins to enjoy her mate's solicitude and this new feeling about the body that she may have paid very little attention to before.

Changing Life Patterns

Getting ready for parenting brings a turnabout in the daily patterns of each individual as well as those patterns evolved as a couple. Old patterns must now be reevaluated. Preparing for the fifteen-hour workdays ahead begins with learning how to conserve energy. Examining the priorities in one's life should take place in the first trimester. By jotting down a list of present priorities it will soon become evident that many changes must take place to accommodate a new baby in the family. Time for relaxation every day should be at the top of the list, although even when time is faithfully set aside to relax the couple should not be dismayed if they cannot, at will, wind their bodies down. With daily practice, the art of relaxation will come in time. Particularly in the infant's early months, setting aside a regular period of time to relax can mitigate the parents' exhaustion.

If the woman has not learned how to schedule her day, she can form new patterns during her months of waiting that will allow her to cope with all the changes her baby will bring. Doing tasks regularly can free time, not only for relaxation, but for completing old projects that, if not finished before the birth, will probably hang around for another couple of years. Eating meals at regular times as well as sleeping at regular times builds energy and gives the pregnant woman time to learn some new skill, to research some subject of interest, to satisfy her creative desires, and to fully prepare for motherhood. When the baby comes, having been on a schedule herself, she will more easily maneuver the infant into a schedule.

Taking short courses in first aid can build a woman's confidence in handling emergencies with infants. What to do if the baby is dropped, swallows something, bumps the head, needs artificial respiration, or is troubled by any of the countless frightening eventualities that might occur in infant care are easily learned skills.

Attending birthing classes together (or with a close friend for the single woman) will help to build confidence in the couple (or the single parent). In the birthing class, the expectant mother will be able to consciously experience labor before it actually takes place. Attending films of birthings can be invaluable for both the man and the woman. To vicariously experience the labor and birth ahead of time, she will have to fully understand the phases of labor and practice the science of breath and the art of relaxation. There are many methods to choose from. A woman's particular method should enable her to be master of her body and to work with pain without fear. Bradley, Lamaze, Leboyer, yogic methods, and other breath-relaxation-prophylaxis techniques are available. Many Sufi women work with the water breath, which is breathing in through the nose and out through the mouth in a four/four rhythm. All of the puffing techniques begin with mastery of the water element breath.

Long-lasting relationships may be formed with friends made at birthing class as well as with other couples with young children as the molding, growing, and strong emotions experienced together at this time proceed. Babies who grow up together aid in forming strong but subtle bonds between their parents.

Keeping a Journal

The weeks of waiting are a perfect time for the woman to cultivate routine journal writing. The process of writing can bring realizations and understanding that would otherwise be only subconscious inklings. Particularly during this time of growth it is valuable for the woman to record her experiences, feelings, changes happening in the relationship, and physical aspects of the pregnancy. It is instructive to read these entries during successive pregnancies. It is also interesting to children to read about situations that happened when their mother was pregnant with them. Reviewing her own childhood experiences with her mother will give stronger recall and more understanding of the phases that her own child will go through. Many of her own childhood experiences will naturally recur as she nurtures and guides her own pregnancy.

When the baby is born it never seems as if there is enough time. The habit of writing in the journal will hopefully continue — for catching special moments with her child, transitions the child goes through, and important experiences that mold the child's perception. The journal can be a priceless tool that will enable the mother to understand in retrospect how events and experiences that at the time had no apparent connection were actually closely related. Later in life this same journal can be a key in helping children to reconstruct their past patterning and to understand their own nature more fully. One example of the importance of journal keeping is when the mother notes the time when the child cuts the first molars. This will give the key to when the child's self-will manifested, as the entries will correlate. Also the pattern of the child's natural development emerges from the mother's entries in the journal.

Parental concepts of freedom, limitations, scheduling, self-discipline, and patterning will change. Through journal writing, parenting goals can begin to be established ahead of time. Particularly if the couple is involved in care of other young infants and toddlers, they will discover enough questions regarding their own parenting goals to help them establish a unified approach.

PSYCHOSPIRITUAL ADJUSTMENT FOR THE EXPECTANT FATHER

The prospective father also experiences a crisis of acceptance. He has the pressing responsibility to work on his own attitudes and goals early in the pregnancy. The body of knowledge he received in his own early childhood can be expected to surface at this time. Good experiences will have provided him with the potential of becoming a solid rock in the stormy seas to come. Early developmental transitions he may not have completed may surface and cause fears and uncertainties as well as temporary shirking of responsibility. Providing for a family and accepting emotional responsibility for the new role as parent and protector may temporarily shake his faith in himself. The lack of positive experiences in his early life and the search for encouragement for his male pride may lead him to seek for his own family roots. Here he may see his own father in a new light and turn again to the ideal he saw in this man at seven years of age. While completing this developmental cycle of transition he may feel that parenting is a difficult crisis to face. This phase is usually followed by an increase in serious thinking and thoughtful decision making, which gives him better control of his emotional and behavioral reactions to fatherhood.

A sense of humor and the motherly understanding of his mate can bring forth new goals for his new role as parent. Observing the relationship between fathers and sons, fathers and daughters, and other couples will also aid him in his own goal-building. "Getting his trip together" in these early months of pregnancy will smooth the transition into fatherhood.

The father's reaction can be so important to the pregnant woman because his expectancy and joy in the coming event aid her in accepting the first trying tests of pregnancy, when excessive physical discomforts and psychological withdrawal may hinder the quickening.

When the man shares in the experience of attending birthing classes, it encourages the sharing of hopes and expectations with other fathers-to-be and erases his own hidden fears. By bringing into the light of consciousness the remembered lacks in fathering during his own earliest childhood, he may be able to set goals and objectives of his own. The connections he makes now with other men in prenatal groups may build friendships that will last for years to come.

This is a time of changing goals and the urge to change jobs and residence. Moves that must be made should be planned in the first trimester. The nest is best transferred with largely male energy. The delivery of the baby is often adversely affected by moving the nest in the last trimester and therefore the father should take responsibility to avoid this error in judgment.

If there are stressful memories of previous miscarriages, the father's comfort and reassurance will aid the mother to move forward with hopeful and happy expectations for the present pregnancy. The father should be patient and understand the mother's preoccupation with past experiences and gently use humor to ease her out of her moods. Through the positive reinforcement in his loving glance he will assure her of his love and admiration for her new look, enjoying the glow and radiance of her burgeoning motherhood.

This is a time for the man to strengthen his emotional body in order that he can be present and supportive at the birth of his child. There are things that only a father can do at the birthing. He will be the first person to hold his child and may whisper the sacred phrase into the child's left ear, thus giving the first impress of the spiritual goal to the soul. He can monitor the bonding of mother and child, the cutting and saving of the cord and placenta, the latter to be planted beneath the child's birthday tree at home, a young tree that will grow as the child grows. He can plan to substitute for the mother in bonding eye to eye with his child, in case of cesarean birth or any other emergency preventing mother-infant bonding. He will plan to follow through on what his mate and he have planned in case of a last-minute change of birthing plans.

SPIRITUAL NUTRITION FOR THE EXPECTANT MOTHER

Not only proper diet, but also emotional tranquility, exercise, fresh air, and a program of spiritual growth will maintain the mother's health and happiness and will facilitate passage through fetal development without mishap. Walking and playing outdoors, exercising regularly, and consciously supplying balanced nutrition to her physical body will become her new standard of living.

Relaxation is a key to an easier birth; the pregnancy will go much smoother if the couple — particularly the woman — focuses on learning it. Relaxation methods are many and varied and may include hatha yoga, swimming, dancing, tai chi, gardening in pots or in the garden, walking on the beach, exercising to music, and tensing and relaxing the muscles from head to foot while lying down or meditating. The woman will want to find the techniques that are fun for her and make them a part of her daily schedule — as important as eating regular meals and snacks and as getting eight hours of sleep and naps. Exchanging hand and foot massages can be a great relaxation at the end of the day.

Attuning to the water element should start as early as pregnancy is confirmed. Activities that help the woman get in touch with the water-element aspect of the pregnancy should be practiced: swimming, bathing leisurely, water massage, taking a dip under a waterfall, concentrating on the water, and doing water-breath practices and mantras. Following her bath or shower with a cold-water massage is an enlivening, rejuvenating practice. Using a loofah sponge to briskly rub the skin in the water is great for the elasticity of the skin and for sloughing off dead cells.

Dancing with other pregnant women gives the expectant mother a creative outlet and good rhythmic exercise, as well.

Many beautiful dances may be created just by interpreting women saints in movement. Imagine these qualities in your own subconscious being and bring them up to the surface in movement and rhythm.

Watch movements in nature, such as the blossoming of flowers, the bending of tall trees against the wind, the billowing sails of sailing ships, the movements of the sylphs in cloud formations, and all the beautiful gestures that the hands may express for the movements of water, fire, and air. Lie close to Mother Earth occasionally, listening to her rhythms and sucking up the good magnetism from her bosom. Walk barefoot on the sands of the beach and on smooth dirt paths. As you do so, inhale that magnetism through the feet and up into the heart, then exhale down the arms and let it flow from your fingers back into Mother Earth. Feel the magnetism through your outstretched fingertips. For thousands of years, women before you have tuned themselves to the elements and have gained strength and courage when their souls felt timid.

All creative and uplifting experiences — such as dancing, singing, playing music, painting, and reading or writing poetry, literature, or humor — send good vibrations into the amniotic fluid, building the personality of the child. The pregnant couple should share some inspiration together every day. Crooning lullabies to the baby in utero has a most wonderful effect on the mother and infant. Instrumental accompaniments are encouraged, but if neither parent plays an instrument, lullaby tapes and records will suffice. Music of the masters and music that the mother-to-be makes herself can gear the emotional and spiritual parts of her nature, lifting her vibrations so that she begins to see new life emerging in all creation. Both mother and father should cultivate their musical abilities, for first inner vibrations and then sounds of the outside world reach and affect the fetus. Through singing comes sharing, which contributes to the relaxation of parents and baby.

A woman will find great reinforcement of her faith and hope through the reading of sacred literature, the purpose of which is not to educate or to intellectually enlighten her mind, but to place her spirit in humble submission and receptivity before creative, inspiring holy beings who serve humanity in exceptional ways. Thus, the secrets of spiritual living are imparted by the mother's concentration, through the subtle bodies, to the fetus. When she reads spiritual literature, the woman will find that the messages she is ready to receive will resound within her and those she is not ready for will pass right through. She should not worry about understanding it all — it is the impress that counts. Years later, she will see manifested in her child the attributes her spiritual reading influenced during pregnancy.

Furthermore, in studying her own religious heritage and further exploring the Divine Mother in comparative religion, the woman can develop the foundations of her own mothering more fully. The early lives of prophets, saints, and masters can broaden and deepen her knowledge and belief in her own sacred mission as the transition into maturity takes place. Some great spiritual works about women, childbearing, purity, and the soul's descent are listed in the Appendix.

The months of pregnancy are a heightened time for understanding the feminine, attuning to nature, and developing creative instincts. Exploring nature literature and making excursions into the animal and bird kingdoms will show the pregnant woman how animals and birds nurture their young and will strengthen her understanding of her own role. Some books that are beautifully attuned to nature are also listed in the Appendix, as are nonfiction books and novels that deal with the feminine and nature.

QUICKENING

Quickening is when the mother feels fetal movement for the first time, as a fluttering within the womb, which sometimes produces faintness. It occurs in the fourth month and affects all women differently. In the early part of the first trimester, the period of pregnancy where the mother may not be aware or sure that the conception has taken place, an electric blue light appears to those who are psychically or mystically inclined. It can be seen glowing cloudlike over the navel of the mother. As soon as the quickening takes place, there is a separate will and movement of the fetus, independent from the mother, to which she must submit. At this time, there is a tremendous change in the energy field or spirit of that soul outside of the mother's body; it is quite obvious to those who witness phenomena that the light over the navel begins to spin after quickening. In understanding what is happening during this period it is important to realize that there are five systems developing, each at its own rate, although they sometimes overlap or hesitate, creating energy manifestations that change rapidly.

In the fourth month the spiritual body of the expectant mother expands; she is acutely sensitive at this time — more so than at any time other than the hours of delivery. This is why abortion in this month hinders spiritual development for years to come. No one has yet discovered how to sever the psychic umbilical cord when new life is aborted. An insult is given to the emotional body of the woman that heals very slowly.

The quickening ushers in a period of subconscious fantasizing for the woman and what appears to her family to be moody, imaginative "trips" (indulgence). Actually, she is beginning to adjust herself, psychically, emotionally, and spiritually, to the new being. Through her first act of self-renunciation she extends herself into the personality and the being of this new entity growing within her womb. She then realizes that one part of her is battling to hold her own, while another part is making every effort to reach and attune to the fetus, to nourish and consciously feed its efforts to attain the integration of its body — skeletal, muscular, nervous, lymph, circulatory, digestive, excretory, respiratory, endocrinal, and reproductive systems as well as the mental, emotional, spiritual, and social bodies — all at an unbelievable pace.

In this second phase, the fetus now dominates the mother's physical body, attempting to master her will through its patterns of behavior — kicking and turning, affecting her body chemistry, and demonstrating its other remarkable powers. The fetus has at last become a reality to the mother because it moves and turns and has a will of its own; it does not always turn when she would want it to, it kicks when she would not have it kick, and it sometimes gives her restless nights. Often during these times that are meant for the mother's rest and sleep, it seems that the fetus becomes the most active. This separate personality thus manifests in a way that demands recognition. At this great moment in fetal life, the mother recognizes the child, for the first time, as a separate yet attached extension of herself. This realization is the first preparation for the physical separation of the infant from her body at birth.

Surprisingly enough, our culture has no prescribed antidotes for the inner turmoil that inevitably follows the quickening. In older cultures, however, accommodation for this experience is always made. In Thailand, the mother-to-be purchases a little earthen statue of a mother image holding an infant to her heart, which she wears until the baby is born. It is then thrown into the river, where its unfired clay melts away in the running waters.

Some African tribal witch doctors prepare the image that the mother will wear around her neck until the birth. These ancient and symbolic rituals centering around the quickening experience enable the mother to sever the "psychic umbilical cord" by her own will when the time comes. The fetus's independent movements and will are symbolically severed from the mother before birth takes place. There is much to be said for these ancient rituals that pave the way for teaching mothers that they do not possess their sons and daughters forever, nor may they keep them "tied to their apron strings" into adult life, as do many unfulfilled married women, widows, and single parents in our culture.

The quickening seems to cause the young mother to enter a mentally active period, when the possible personality and attributes of her baby tantalize her. The fear that her child may inherit her worst qualities may torment her. Fears that the baby may be abnormal or that one of the different fetal developmental changes might go awry also may irk her. Her mind wanders as she wonders. This pondering can be understood as the divine force working within her mind, forcing her to reorganize her thinking to adjust to her new role as guide to her child. It is also a period when the intuitive faculties enable her to attune to her infant's movements, surmising its individual need for exercise. The infant's kicking and pressures demand changing old patterns of resting and sleeping.

QUICKENING AFFECTS EXPECTANT FATHERS DEEPLY

The quickening experience is shared by the father and starts the bonding between him and his child. By laying his hands on her belly and gently massaging clockwise toward the navel he will thrill to the first movements of his child. Through sharing their discoveries of the personality and spirit of their child, the couple will also confide their concerns and mutually reassure each other. The fears of pregnancy will soon be softened and eased. As they meditate together, sharing the closeness of the great servers of humanity they have read about, the commitment to their child will increase.

It is important that the stage be set for the father early in pregnancy. Now he is ready to turn to the real work of his pregnant mate. First he must listen, *really listen*, to the inner guidance the mother-to-be is receiving, which she will often doubt. In listening to her and tuning in to her doubtful moments he can reinforce her faith in herself. The changes that pregnancy brings will hinder her from doing many of the physical tasks she used to perform with ease. The father must be sensitive and aware so that he will be able to monitor her desires to do the things she is no longer capable of doing. The lifting, carrying, and pushing tasks must now be set aside for others to perform.

Through all of the changes that the pregnant woman experiences, the father-to-be must maintain the quality of a rock, standing firm and dependable — consoling, flattering, reflecting the vision of the beauty of his Madonna back to her eyes through the mantle of love with which he may now surround her. To be a rock in a time of emotional transition, the father will need to maintain his spiritual practices faithfully, often in silence while his work in the world goes on. The quality of the rock is one of softness to the touch and firmness within. A rock can roll with the emotional and mental upheavals the mother-to-be goes through as her body chemistry changes while he maintains his own emotional strength. In becoming a firm foundation for his family, he also becomes the point of reference for the security of his mate and child.

Once the man has accepted his role, he must consider this as a most sacred trust, one in which he pledges to give himself to his child, secure in the faith that he will receive back two-fold from the Spirit of Guidance (the Holy Spirit) the best of his nature. His own guardians are ever present to assist him in the moments when human strength and will fail. The fetus his mate carries within her is still largely functioning on the angelic planes. It, too, is undergoing great and marvelously intricate changes and adjustments to our earth plane as the spirit, en route through the djinn plane, gathers the impress of its soul purpose — bringing with it from those higher planes the many octaves of the chromosomal pairs that we find in the physical pattern. Infancy is the time when the negative soul qualities are becoming positive. So the father or father-image must be a positive influence on the child who enters the environment that both parents have lovingly built; fresh, untired, enthusiastic, and tuned to the years ahead. "The higher the spiritual development of a person the greater the impressions that come from him; the more lasting, the more effective."[1]

The spiritual community can also support the expectant father's needs. Working harder to advance his present goals by completing his education or by planning to go into business with a spiritual brother may also extend his horizons. The interest of the spiritual community in welcoming and making accommodation for the infant aids the man with his transition into parenting. The couple may discuss with close friends their desire to have them present at the birthing. Others may plan a feast to follow the birthing, which the father may host. Gifts of the spirit are the greatest reinforcement to the young father at this time of euphoric thankfulness.

1. Simone de Beauvoir interview.

CHAPTER FIVE

Spiritual Guidance in Pregnancy

Mothering invites the habit of prayer for prayer is a natural builder of self-confidence in caretaking. Anxiety over the great responsibility of nurturing and protecting the development of the fetus is lessened by prayer. Faith in divine guidance, which is built by talking to God within the heart, builds self-confidence and emotional security. Prayer that begins with glorification leads to stress-dissipating good thoughts. Prayer is a great relaxation technique. It controls fear and anxiety by allowing the free flow of mind and heart.

By placing her open hands across her belly and feeling at one with the fetus, the mother can share her innermost feelings and thoughts by means of transferring the electromagnetic field through her palms. By pulling down the light of the Spirit of Guidance through her fontanel and directing it to her heart the mother begins the spiritual bonding by means of her breath and her magnetism. "Talking to the baby" at this early stage of development impresses nerve ganglia through the power of thought-form.

The full implications of becoming a spiritual guide to her child demand contact with a higher Being to support the mother in relinquishing the psychic hold on the baby — somehow thinking of the baby as a possession. Her divine duty is to nurture and guide that soul and spirit during the time previous to birth, to be caretaker, not possessor.

Prayer reinforces supportive attitudes in that it brings into harmony the mother's fantasies and her quickly changing feelings about her new role and its future evolution. Becoming conscious of the fetal movements during prayer awakens her to the reality of the effect of her own body drives, emotional states, and spritual "highs" on the fetus. Through the practice of daily prayer, she can gain inner guidance, added protection, and control over her own needs and fulfillments. Purification of the mind and spirit are the fruits of prayer. In laying firm foundations in her prayer life, the mother can assure the means of keeping contact when her children leave the nest years later. A sense of fulfillment and purpose enters her being, which makes every pregnant woman a beautiful Madonna to the seeing world.

As the Divine Mother principle begins to operate within her heart, the mother feels delight in her fertility. The universal experience of childbearing, with its many sacrifices and joys, leads to a very sacred and intimate relationship between fetus and mother. Through prayer she grows with the fetus, extending her consciousness into the angelic spheres as she grounds herself to Mother Earth in her nature walks. The continuity of life and the hope of extending her being through the generations is explored, enlarged, and built into true concepts of what spiritual growth through prayer really means. To be able to communicate with the God within bridges and heals the weaknesses in her own character. Ever so gently the woman separates from her old single self, becoming one with the new identity, pledging her patience, love, and understanding. Some acts of self-offering aid in this commitment. The following practices are suggested to aid women in getting through the first test of pregnancy.

The mother-to-be may begin her act of adoration upon awakening each morning. Dissolving self-love into mother-love is the initiation into the creation of new life. Just as no two parents can possibly predict or know before birth the kind of child they have made, they cannot foresee the consequences of their commitment to guide and to guard the new life they are responsible for bringing into the world. Learning to pray to the God within in the earliest stages of pregnancy builds a foundation of strength in repeated acts of devotion.

In offering herself to the will of God, as Mary. did when the angel Gabriel announced her pregnancy, she surrenders her own plans and schemes and places the new life in God's hands, accepting any kind of a soul He will send, with joy and faith. She might repeat in prayer, "Enable me to serve Thy Divine Purpose." Next, the mother-to-be learns to daily offer her husband or mate and the life purpose of her unborn child to the Divine Purpose, reminding herself that both belong first to God and only secondly to her.

As Mary, the mother of Jesus, could not foresee that thirty years later this precious life would be hanging on a cross, so the spiritual mother-to-be must offer up this gift of God uncalculatingly, unconditionally, asking nothing in return but to be a devoted guide, whatever the future may hold. When she has decided, in full consciousness, to carry through this pregnancy she is likely to realize the truth of her womanhood — that it is indeed more blessed to give than to receive. With this decision will come deep and abiding joy, peace, and power in her new role.

She may act as Divine Mother toward her mate in her new sexual role by finding new ways of expressing her love through fingertip massage and caressing. Her growing enjoyment of her whole new presence and the firm fullness of breasts and belly tend to make her see herself as a full woman and to reflect that image to her mate.

As each new physical change takes place within the body, she may accept it as coming from the providence and care of God. By building early the habit of relating all physical changes of her pregnancy to God, she will learn to see her child's development in His Light. This early attitude of mind cures anxiety, worry, and fear. When she accepts all that is happening to her body and emotions as coming from God, she learns the secret of living in the now, freed from her own past and her child's unknown future. Right now is hers. Her past and her future belong to God.

At bedtime, she may lie in the corpse position (flat on her back, arms at sides, palms up) and quietly review the day before the Divine Beloved. With thankfulness and with a prayer of self-offering as the child's first guide, she may go to sleep with the guide's prayer on her lips:

> Beloved Lord, Almighty God,
> Through the chain of all masters and saints,
> Through the guides of all angels and children,
> Place my feet firmly on the path of Light,
> Illuminate my mind, purify my heart, and make me a
> Clear channel to my child.[1]

Doing spiritual practices on a regular basis brings a deepened sense of the Divine Presence in all of the events she passes through. It is likely to convince her that all events happen through God and in God and contain only blessings for new family unity. As the first guide practices subjugating her desires and self-wishes to the presence of God, integrating the experience into the fulfillment of motherhood, the small desires of self-will wither and fade. The first test and challenge of this crisis will pass as self-love and love for the new entity come to terms with each other.

During the first trimester, when morning sickness may appear, the mother's physical body and her will not to be mastered by the entity will be challenged. The physical symptoms of heartburn, morning sickness, and flatulence, which admittedly can be unpleasant, are often due to changes in the body chemistry, and nutritionists advise adding magnesium and vitamin B-6 to the diet to help overcome this annoyance.

If she awakens to nausea, she will be strengthened each morning if she uses this time of enforced stillness in bed to develop the spiritual practice of intercession. For example, she can recite the Lord's Prayer in this manner:

Our Father, which art in the Heaven within me,
Thy name be hallowed within my child.
Thy Kingdom come into my womb,
Thy Will be done in my child's growth,
As it is done in Thy angelic heaven.
Give my child its daily spiritual food,
Forgive today its soul's past trespasses,
And lead its soul to forgive those who trespassed
     against it on other planes.
Lead its life away from temptations,
And deliver it safely into our world.[2]

As she realizes what it means to prepare herself for mothering, the meditation of going into the uterus and "seeing" the growth of the child will enable her to begin to forget herself. Instead of fighting the physical changes and unpleasant side effects, she may find a transformation taking place within her, reflected outwardly in Madonna-like beauty, compassion, love, and charity toward all children.

Through the mother's prayer and constancy, impressions, visions, or dreams may clarify the soul purpose of the entity and make known the name of the child. The father often receives this. A vision of the entity — the type of child she is to bear, its character, and personality — may begin to manifest to her. Through prayer she also faces all the fears of abnormalities that occur to every pregnant woman at some time in the pregnancy. In the third trimester, the mother's intuition is likely to become highly active. Knowing the soul's attributes — positive or negative, aggressive or peaceful — may disturb her mental body. This turmoil can be calmed by reading aloud spiritually inspiring literature each day. Preparing her heart for mothering brings tranquility. The expectant mother may say:

Beloved Lord, behold Thy child _____.
Beloved Lord, I offer Thee this my desire for _____.
Thy will be done in his/her life.

This prayer can spiritually change the mother's will and can clarify God's purpose. Recognizing how God uses her daily for her child's growth can create a healing physical environment.

Even in the first twenty weeks of pregnancy, the mental/emotional makeup of the child is being determined. This is a good time for the mother to begin conscious concentration and meditation on the developing embryo and the divine plan in earnest. A conscious pregnancy is a pregnancy in which the mother is aware of the stages of development within the womb from conception onward and in which she mentally and inwardly tunes to the wonder of creation going on within her body. Conscious pregnancy is also putting to work her own five bodies — physical, mental, emotional, spiritual, and social — to imprint her child. Conscious pregnancies often culminate in births of full-term, healthy babies as well as in consciousness and awareness of the initiation into motherhood.

The mother must realize that the human fetus reacts to the emotional and physical traumas that she allows herself to go through. Acts of God — death in the family, accidents, or sudden shocks — may not be avoidable but the reaction to them can certainly be mitigated by practicing positive affirmation, silence, and meditation, all of which will build inner security.

The heart expansion into this consciousness can open the mother to a new sensitivity. She may see herself reflecting the attitudes and behavior of those about her and picking up thoughts from other people. The realization that thought-forms are as real to her now as the spoken word used to be enables her to gain wisdom and peace of mind. Pregnancy stimulates her new awareness of self, rewarding and urging her to be choosy about her associates and surroundings.

FETAL DEVELOPMENT

The mother can develop an understanding of the changes the fetus is undergoing by keeping a monthly chart of the developmental progress of the fetus. This will aid her concentration and in turn affect the fetal development in a positive way.

It is amazing to realize how much is happening as early as the third week. The embryo is two millimeters long and already has a brain divided into three main sections. The heart tube is beating, the inner ear is forming, and the retinas and optic nerves are forming in the eyes. The placenta is starting to grow and all systems (except the musculoskeletal and reproductive systems) have at least developed cells that are ready to be organized to accomplish their destined function. Being aware of the effect that her conscious mental and emotional attitudes have on the fetus aids the mother in gaining wisdom and mastery of nature's processes in utero. It is possible in the first trimester to become acquainted with the type of soul the couple has attracted.

As for the incoming soul, it must patiently await its housing while the delicate first trimester of pregnancy determines whether it will stay or delay. The second trimester will build confidence and security in the incarnating soul and the third trimester will culminate in birth — the inhaling of the first breath, which carries the soul into captivity for this life span. Just as the djinn-plane inhabitants give impress to the soul's new life purpose, so do the mother's intake of food and breath, her blood circulation, and her joys and traumatic experiences (physical and emotional) influence the physical impress and the physical limitations the soul must master.

Developmental Visualization

Being involved with a strong new soul of quite different energy than her own may at first frighten, then surprise, and finally demand acceptance of her. Likewise, a gentle soul coming to a strong, energetic mother may cause her to feel taken aback, slowed down, and forced to change her rhythm. Contemplation and meditation can be of great comfort at this time, clarifying and often manifesting the being who has chosen to embody through her. A method that works well in bringing about the accommodation for the new soul without losing self-identity is to follow in meditation the development of the baby from fetus to a fully developed baby. During the period when the heart is forming, the mother-to-be can do the heart concentration. During the development of the eyes, she can concentrate on that, and so forth. Each month she focuses on that aspect of the fetus where the most growth is taking place. By using her own insight she can build a strong mental image of the little embryo in light. A monthly concentration on the stages of fetal development along with a chart of growth for the mother to focus on daily are presented below.

The following visualizations and concentrations on each stage of development were first used in my own pregnancies many years ago and were subsequently refined and coordinated with the teachings of Hazrat Inayat Khan, the Vedic teachings, and modern astrology. These concentrations are important as a tool for spiritual women to become consciously aware of the mysteries within conception and birth and attuned to the wonder of human development. The Sufi rose, the talisman, has been used as an ancient symbol of beauty to focus the pregnant woman's concentration upon the important alchemical process taking place in utero. The Divine Being associated with each month expands the consciousness of the expectant mother by putting her in touch with the prototypes within her own being.

Before beginning, hold palms of both hands over belly. Next, (1) study each detail of the illustration, (2) stare fixedly for sixty seconds at the picture of the fetus, (3) close your eyes, pick up the image in your inner eye, and transfer it to the fetus. Lose yourself in the presence of the angels, masters, saints, and prophets as they come through.

Contemplation precedes concentration. Concentration precedes meditation. The eye focuses in and the mind builds its own image. The meditation places you in contact with the hierarchy of angels, archangels, kingdoms, and principalities, reflecting the planes of manifestation through which the spirit and soul will evolve and which will become your own particular baby's personality.

Contemplation should happen early in the day, "when the

dew is still on the rose." Concentration follows naturally as the heart tunes to the image of the fetus growing from tight green bud to full-blown rose — the perfection of the seed and sperm brought to perfect fruition. A regular set time for meditation in nature is suggested. Once the practice is established, the time spent practicing is not as important as the experience of being a conscious part of transmitting love and energy to the developing fetus — creating the perfect physical housing for the soul the love experience has attracted.

Some fathers have described the mandalas that they have received during the period when the mothers are doing their concentrations. Jung discovered in his exploration of the collective unconscious that all aboriginal people have the ability to close their eyes and pick up their mandala without effort.[3] This ability may come from the racial memory built into the pineal gland. The inner eye via the psyche would receive the image. Older cultures seem to have the ancestors and prototypes built into their psyche, for almost all find it a natural phenomenon to observe the mandala in meditation.

In Western civilization, we have to work hard for this vision, although young children (beginning at the chronological age of three) at Sufi Seed Centers, can attain this vision, given basic-form concentrations and puzzles. They put together, then contemplate, concentrate, and finally (in silence) pick up the image in the inner eye, which follows their fixed gaze.

The very young child is able to pick up that image quickly, within three to four weeks, without effort. However, it is not clear whether Caucasians, as a race, always had this potential ability or whether they once had use of it and later lost it. It is likely that the Caucasian race has the latent capacity, but that it has never been developed in the Western world, due to hurry, focus on material things, and the lack of basic tranquility that besets the American way of life. At least during pregnancy, however, some women want to reach the realms of Light to usher in the soul. Fathers may pick up the mandala at this time because this is when the genetic inheritance of both parents begins its development within the central nervous system of the fetus.

A few notes about fetal developmental stages will aid the mother-to-be in her understanding. The human develops from the head downward; we learn to grasp before we can walk. The first two months are the embryonic stage, after this the embryo becomes a fetus. In developmental terms, this means that all systems and organs that will be functioning in the adult human have been formed to some degree after the second month. The subsequent months of pregnancy further develop and perfect each organ or system. The greatest period of growth is between the third and fourth months. If born prematurely, a seven-month-old fetus can survive, although an eight-month-old fetus has a far greater chance of survival. All the neurons in the brain are developed by the last weeks of pregnancy, and thereafter increase only in size. At this point, new cells replace the old ones but no increase in the number of cells occurs. Other relevant facts about the fetus at this late point in its development are: it sleeps and probably dreams; it drinks more amniotic fluid if sweetened, less if soured; it can be taught to be alerted for something new; and it hiccups and sucks its thumb. At this stage, the mother's awareness and vibration must certainly be felt by the developing human child.

A baby is usually considered to be full-term 280 days from the first day of the last menstrual period, or 256–270 days from conception, or 10 lunar months (of 28 days each), or 40 weeks. There are discrepancies in the embryological literature as to the timing of each developmental occurrence, partly because some systems begin counting from the first day of the last period, and others from the ovulation time. Also because of the two types of monthly systems, it is sometimes unclear whether a certain event occurs toward the end of one month or the beginning of the next. It would have been preferable to follow the lunar months because, for the spiritual woman, attunement to the cycles of the moon are a natural part of womanhood. However, much of the research was based on the other system. Of course, babies come when they are good and ready, anyway — late or early.

It is important to realize that although the period in the womb brings the process of growth and maturation to the various organs and systems of the human body, some aspects are not completed until adulthood. For example, it takes six months after birth for the vocal cords to be mature; the ossification of bones in the feet and hands are not complete until seventeen years of age; the teeth are not completed until the twenty-fourth year of life; the muscles are not mature until the twenty-fifth year for the woman and the sixteenth year for the man; the digestive system may not fully mature until the second year of life; and the ear is not fully functioning until nine years of age in many American children.

Many women may not know they are pregnant in the first month. If pregnancy is not confirmed until the second month, begin with the second month concentration, but read through the first month's concentration and keep in mind the solar system's connection with the embryo.

FIRST MONTH CONCENTRATION: Focus on the planets revolving around the sun. "As above, so below." What has already been in existence in the cosmos now reflects its blueprint for the fetal development through the individual universe being formed on the physical plane. "The soul is light, the mind is light, and the body is light — light of different grades; and it is this relation which connects man with the planets and the stars." 4 Focus on the dominant planet(s) of the sun sign at the time of conception.

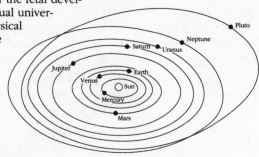

SYMBOL: Our solar system.

HOLY BEING: The Divine Mother,
who is the archetype of all earthly mothers and who exists in all women.

FETAL DEVELOPMENT: All basic organ systems are beginning to form.

AT THE END OF THE FIRST MONTH

SIZE	3/16 inch; 1/140 ounce
NEUROLOGY	The spinal cord has been formed — the primitive brain differentiated from spinal cord. An unmistakable human brain is formed at 30 days — the first organ to begin development.
RESPIRATORY	The placenta has been formed jointly by maternal and embryonic tissue to bring in oxygen and nutrients from the mother and to take carbon dioxide and waste products from the embryo.
DIGESTION	The digestive system is beginning to form, the stomach is distinguishable from the esophagus, and the basic kidneys, liver, pancreas, and gall bladder are formed.
LIMBS	The arm and leg buds are showing.
CIRCULATION	The heart, one of the first organs to develop, has increased greatly in size during this month, but is not complete. Heart pumps blood at end of month. Yolk sac forms blood cells.
FACE AND SENSES	No nose, eyes, or external ears are visible, although they are present by the end of the month. The mouth membrane ruptures in preparation for eventual ingestion.
APPEARANCE	It looks like a fish and has a coiled endpiece that looks like a fishtail. There are folds below the eye spot that are gill formations.
ENDOCRINE SYSTEM	The beginnings of thyroid, anterior pituitary, dorsal and ventral pancreas are now developed.

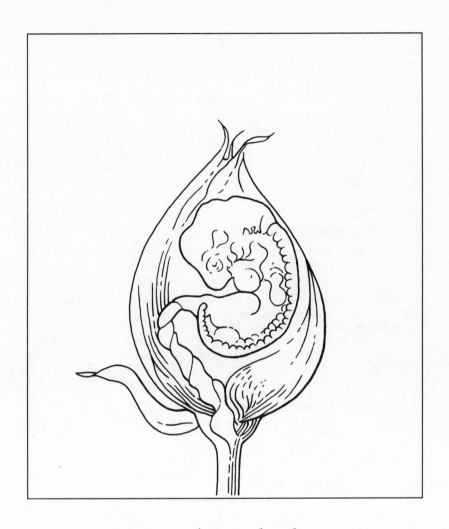

*"Little rosebud,
so tightly closed,
what beauty is hidden
in thy heart?"* [5]

SECOND MONTH CONCENTRATION: Focus on the rays of the Divine Light coming into your heart. Pick up the one ray your child's soul is entering on and envision your cherub. "May the rays of the Divine Sun shining in Thy heart be reflected in the hearts of Thy devotees."[6]

SYMBOL: Star of the Divine Light — the beginning of life.

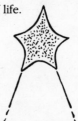

HOLY BEING: Archangel Auriel — the Divine Light of God.

FETAL DEVELOPMENT: Pawlike, or webbed hands and feet are forming. The five points of the star symbol relates to the five webbed fingers.

AT THE END OF THE SECOND MONTH

SIZE	1-1/8 inch; 1/30 ounce
NEUROLOGY	The developing cerebral hemispheres show through the transparent skin. The ear, eye, and nose nerves connect with the brain. Brain waves can be detected at 45 days.
RESPIRATORY	Lung cavities are separated by the diaphragm. The gill arches disappear as the lungs begin their function of sucking in the amniotic fluid.
DIGESTION	A distinct umbilical cord is formed.
LIMBS	Limbs begin to differentiate into arm, elbows, forearm, and hand; thigh, knee, lower leg, and foot. Pawlike hands and webbed feet form.
CIRCULATION	The liver of the fetus produces its own blood as the yolk sac decreases in size and function. The circulation system for the brain is complete.
FACE	The dark eye spot can be seen. Eyelids are folds above the eye spot. Facial features are beginning to form — the upper lid is completed, the nose is more prominent, and there is a hole for the ear.
APPEARANCE	The tail-like part of the embryo disappears. The head is half the size of the body, and not so bent over.
INTERNAL	Long bones and internal organs are developing.
SKELETAL	The skeleton is complete in cartilage formation in 45 days. Buds of teeth appear.
MOVEMENT	From 7-1/2 to 9-1/2 weeks, total involuntary body movements begin.
SEXUALITY	Male and female look alike.

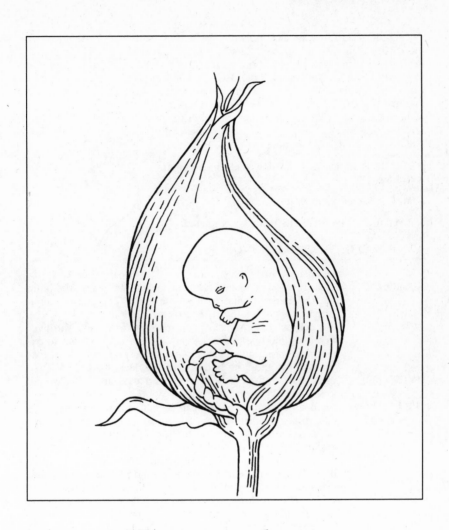

*"Flowers, speak to me
of Thy loveliness, and
tell me how beautiful
Thou art."* [7]

THIRD MONTH CONCENTRATION: Focus on the responsive heart receiving the Divine Light, liberating itself. Renounce all selfish desires and extend your heart to meet the pure heart of your angel child. Listen to the heartbeat of the fetus with a stethoscope, if possible. Hold pointer and middle fingers to right side of your windpipe. Close eyes and listen for your own heartbeat. Breathe on that rhythm as you concentrate on bringing the Light of God down through your crown center to your heart, then to the heart of the fetus. Begin and end the day doing this. Five minutes at a time is enough.

HOLY BEING: Jesus, with the sacred heart aflame with love.

SYMBOL: Sacred heart of Jesus.

FETAL DEVELOPMENT: The heart is completed.

AT THE END OF THE THIRD MONTH

SIZE	3 inches; 1 ounce
NEUROLOGY	Special regions and structures are developed within the brain (such as neural connections to the ear). The cerebral hemispheres are ballooning. The fetus feels pain.
DIGESTION	The cells of the stomach begin to secrete mucus. The liver secretes some bile into intestines and the kidneys start to expel urine into amniotic fluid — just for practice. The throat can swallow and taste buds are highly developed.
LIMBS	Arms, hands, fingers, legs, feet, and toes are fully formed now and nails begin to develop.
CIRCULATION	The heart is completed and can be detected with special fetal heart monitor instruments. The beats are usually between 140 and 170 beats per minute. The first truly mature blood cells are being formed.
FACE	The eyes are almost fully developed. The eyelids meet and fuse. The external ear is present. Sound reaches the ear, but no emotional response is noted. Mouth, nose, and throat are extensively developed. The lips move in a sucking motion. The face can squint, frown, or look surprised.
APPEARANCE	The head is extended and the neck lengthened. True skin has now replaced the first protective membrane. The fetus becomes individualized, and has outer facial expression.
INTERNAL	Within the hardening jaw all 20 tooth buds appear. Cartilage centers change into bone and neuromuscular coordinators.
MOVEMENT	The facial muscles are moving preparatory to rooting and suckling at birth. The mother may feel the baby fluttering from spontaneous movement of arms and legs (quickening).
SEXUALITY	Sex is distinguishable. The male sexual system develops. The female sexual system remains undifferentiated.

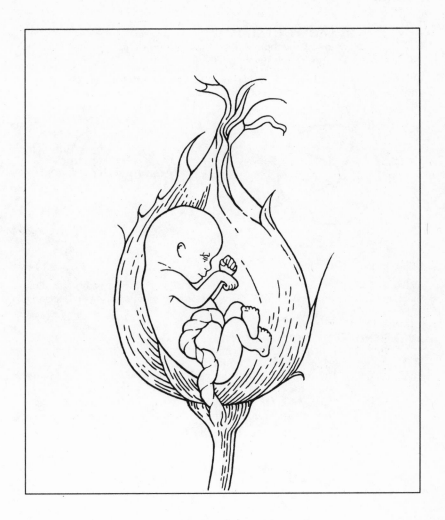

*"My heart,
gather thyself together
as the rose holds
its petals."* [8]

FOURTH MONTH CONCENTRATION: Focus on the spiral which is the symbol of growth. Spinning symbolizes the bringing forth of life. "It is the twist of thought that is the curl of the Beloved." 9

SYMBOL: A whorl made by the Mayas in Central America. It represents God and the universe in perpetual motion.

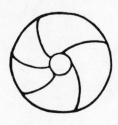 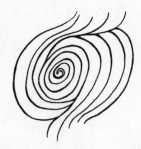

HOLY BEING: Saint Michael, greatest of all archangels.

FETAL DEVELOPMENT: Whorls of hair appear all over the fetus' body, called "lanugo." Quickening occurs; the mother feels fetal movements — the stirring of life.

AT THE END OF THE FOURTH MONTH

SIZE	6-1/2 to 7 inches; 4 ounces
RESPIRATORY	The fetal chest walls move and amniotic fluid moves in and out of the trachea.
DIGESTION	Digestion is fairly efficient. The fetus swallows and urinates.
LIMBS	Touch pads at finger- and toe-tips and at base of digits have developed, but will change to become the individual's unique fingerprints. All joints are complete.
CIRCULATION	A strong heartbeat can be monitored. Blood is now formed by bone marrow instead of by the liver.
FACE	Ears, eyes, nose, and mouth are now of almost typical newborn appearance. Lips, especially the upper lip, protrude. The nostrils are plugged. Eyebrows appear. The palate fuses and vocal cords are mostly complete.
APPEARANCE	The head is one third of body length. The skin appears to be bright red but is actually translucent, showing blood underneath. The entire body is beginning to be covered with downy, soft, fine hair (lanugo) in whorls. Nipples appear. The back becomes straight.
INTERNAL	Most bones are distinctly indicated. Ribs are easy to see.
MOVEMENT	The muscles are active, stretching arms and legs. The fetus is more active when the woman is quiet.
SEXUALITY	The female sexual system differentiates.

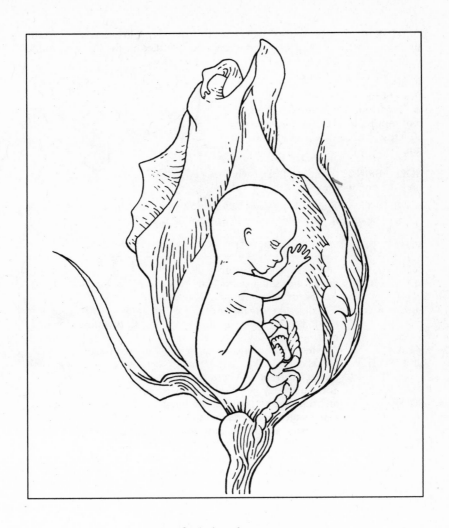

*"Unfold Thy secret
through nature, and reveal
Thy mystery through
my heart."* [10]

FIFTH MONTH CONCENTRATION: Focus on the divine breath of God — the life force within the fetus. Envision your baby cradled in the crescent moon — your receptive heart.

SYMBOL: The divine child in the crescent moon. It is important for you to draw your own symbol. The crescent represents the responsiveness of the crescent moon to the light of the sun.

HOLY BEING: Saint Gabriel, who gave the annunciation to Mary.

FETAL DEVELOPMENT: Lungs and outer skin tissue are developing. The fetus can see, hear, feel, and learn at a primary level in utero.[11]

AT THE END OF THE FIFTH MONTH

SIZE	10 to 12 inches; 8 ounces
RESPIRATORY	Lungs are still insufficiently developed to function outside the uterus.
DIGESTION	The digestive organs are formed but are not ready to take in food. The mother may feel hiccuping (a rhythmic vibration) this month.
LIMBS	The fetus has a reflex; opposed thumb, and finger grip.
CIRCULATION	Heartbeat is 120 to 160, heard by stethoscope but there is no longer need for specialized instruments.
FACE AND SENSES	Some hair may be forming on head and eyebrows. Eyelids are still fused. The ears of the fetus are functioning now. Since water conducts sound better than air does, and since there is no air in the eardrum of the fetus, as there is in the adult human when in water, the fetus hears constant sound — the mother's voice, stomach rumbling, others' voices, radio, and television. (Watch what you view and say.)
APPEARANCE	Bright red, wrinkled skin still persists. The protective creamy vernix is beginning to deposit on the skin and will be absorbed into the skin after birth. The appendages of the evolutionary past, such as the tail, recede this month.
INTERNAL	The internal organs mature at a rapid rate.
MOVEMENT	The fetus may be sucking the thumb, scratching the face, or grasping the umbilical cord. Stroking of the fetal lips produces a protrusion of the lips. The fetus moves in body rhythm to the mother's speech and singing patterns, whether joyous, sad, excited, angry, or peaceful and devotional. The rhythm of music affects the fetal movements. Beethoven makes the fetus kick, Vivaldi relaxes, and Brahms rocks and rolls the fetus back and forth.[12]

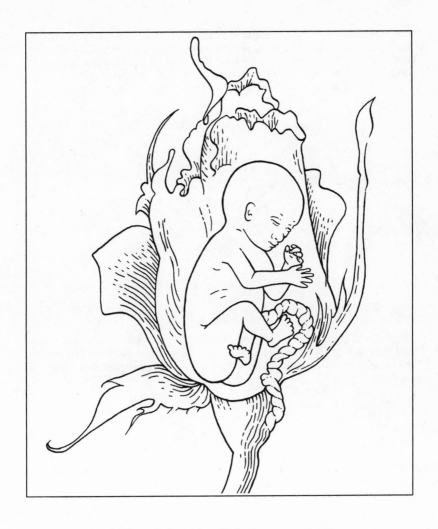

*"The 'lift' which brings a soul
down and takes it back to heaven is
situated within; that 'lift' is the breath;
the soul comes to earth with the breath,
and with the same breath returns."* [13]

SIXTH MONTH CONCENTRATION: Focus on the perfect divine image reflected in the infant — Yahweh, the all-seeing, perfect creator. As the eyelids of the infant open, may the Divine Light shine forth. Meditate upon the virtues you wish to see develop in your child. "The soul of every individual is God, but man has a mind and a body which contain God according to the accommodation."[14]

SYMBOL:

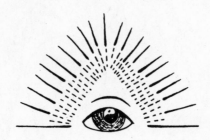

HOLY BEING: Melchizedek, prince of peace, angel of celestial virtues of great grace.

FETAL DEVELOPMENT: The eyelids separate, eyes open, though there is no real sight yet due to membrane. Eyelashes show. Fetus listens all the time to the maternal heartbeat and the father's voice. Audial bonding begins in utero.[15]

AT THE END OF THE SIXTH MONTH

SIZE	11 to 14 inches; 1-1/4 to 1-1/2 pounds
DIGESTION	Pasty, dark green bile, mucus, and dead cells (called meconium) line digestive tract and will be expelled right after the birth, unless a birth trauma ensues, in which case it may be expelled in utero.
LIMBS	Fingernails now extend to the ends of the fingers.
FACE AND SENSES	Eyelids separate and eyelashes form. Membrane covers the pupils, and there is no sight yet.
APPEARANCE	The skin is still somewhat reddish, wrinkled, and covered with vernix caseosa. The skin develops sweat and oil glands and tactile cells that are sensitive to heat, pressure, and pain.
INTERNAL	The skeletal growth is very active up until birth — the mother needs a maximum amount of calcium and magnesium now.
MOVEMENT	Strong arm and leg muscles develop. If the foot is tickled, it plants itself downward (step reflex). At twenty-five weeks, the fetus jumps to drumbeats.[16]

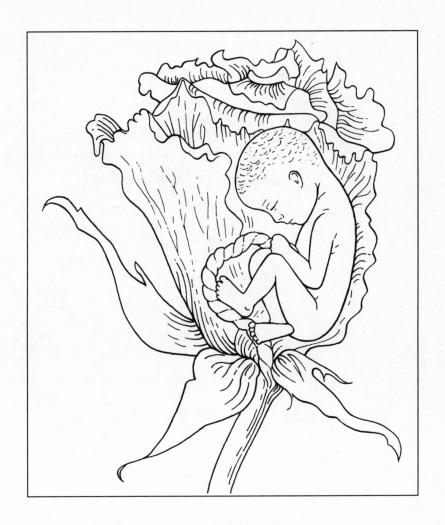

*"Why
have I two eyes
if not to behold Thy
glorious vision?"* 17

SEVENTH MONTH CONCENTRATION: Focus on the Divine Light. Meditate upon the new soul, bringing Light into your life. Idealize the positive traits of character in yourself and your mate. Build a strong self-image of yourself as guide and protector of the new soul. "Pour upon me Thy Love and Thy Light."[18] Look at the solar system representation in the first month concentration. Focus on the planet that will be dominant at the expected time of birth (the planet that rules your child's sun sign).

SYMBOL: The Divine Light, symbolized in the flat-topped triangle that brings the light down to earth.

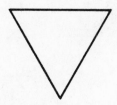

HOLY BEING: Archangel Rafael, one of the watchers, one of the four presences who watch over the diseased and wounded children of humankind. Saint Rafael aids the mother in purifying her mind of all wounds of the heart and all fears.

FETAL DEVELOPMENT: The child receives the Light. True consciousness develops.

AT THE END OF THE SEVENTH MONTH

SIZE	15 inches; 2-1/2 pounds
NEUROLOGY	Convolutions appear in the brain.
RESPIRATORY	The lungs can function minimally outside the uterus (if the baby is born premature), even though they are not yet fully developed.
DIGESTION	The fetus swallows and is able to taste sweet and sour.
FACE AND SENSES	Eyelids open, and the membrane is gone. The eye can receive light (e.g., sunlight on the mother's stomach) and fetus will turn away from bright light. Reaction to sound begins.
APPEARANCE	The skin is like before, still wrinkled and reddish.
SEXUALITY	The male testes descend into the scrotum.
IMMUNE SYSTEM	Antibodies of the mother's immune system can be transmitted between mother and fetus in the last trimester, giving the infant immunity in the first few months (as does breast-feeding).

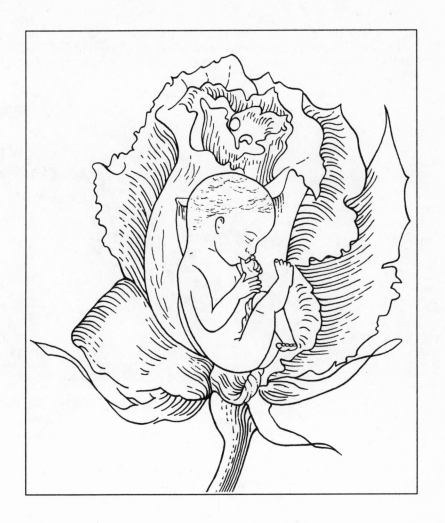

"Rose,
in thy petals
I see the rosy cheeks
of my Beloved." [19]

EIGHTH MONTH CONCENTRATION: Focus on yourself, the woman as the spiritual guide, mediating between the soul of the world and the ideas of mankind. See yourself as guide to the new soul, your mate, and the extended family.

SYMBOL: Twelve-pointed star in a circle, which is the Amish symbol for wisdom.

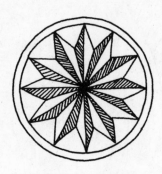

HOLY BEING: Pistis Sophia, wisdom, mother of superior angels. "Wisdom is love and love is true wisdom."[20]

FETAL DEVELOPMENT: The consciousness of the child is developing.

AT THE END OF THE EIGHTH MONTH

SIZE	16-1/2 inches; 4 pounds
NEUROLOGY	The consciousness of the child is developing. At 28 to 32 weeks, the fetal brain neural circuits equal those of the newborn.
LIMBS	The fingers and toes begin to have well-developed nails.
RESPIRATORY	The lungs are much stronger than last month.
DIGESTION	Soft stroking of the cheek produces the characteristic rooting and sucking reflex.
FACE	The bones of the head are soft and flexible.
APPEARANCE	The skin is now more pink and completely covered with vernix. Lanugo begins to disappear. Subcutaneous fat begins to develop, causing the fetus to begin to lose its wrinkled appearance.

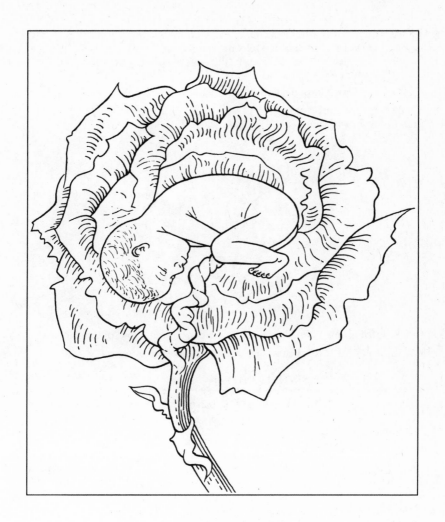

"Rosebud,
what didst thou do all night?
With folded hands I was praying
to heaven to open my heart." [21]

NINTH MONTH CONCENTRATION: Focus on the visualization of a perfectly formed physical body ready to welcome the soul as its occupant with the first breath of life. Meditate on the cherub (the angelic being) coming to you from the realms of Light.

"Toward the One, the perfection of love."

SYMBOL: The cherub coming from the realms of Light.

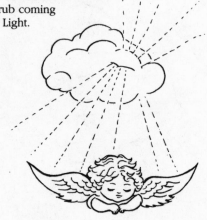

HOLY BEING: Angel Phul, angel of the waters, supreme lord of the waters.

FETAL DEVELOPMENT: Fetus is preparing to leave the womb.

AT THE END OF THE NINTH MONTH

SIZE	19–21 inches long; 6–7-1/2 pounds (10 pounds is still a big baby in the eighties.)
RESPIRATORY	The lungs are self-sufficient.
LIMBS	The fingernails are completed and may protrude beyond the end of the fingers.
CIRCULATION	The placenta begins to become tough and fibrous and does not channel blood like it did before, preparing to force the baby out by decreasing the amount of oxygen.
SENSES	All sense organs are well-formed.
APPEARANCE	The umbilicus is almost in the middle of the body instead of being at the lower end as it was at first. Lanugo usually disappears by now (although some babies are born with it, in which case the parents massage it into the infant's skin at birth). Wrinkles disappear. The soft area (fontanel) above the forehead is shaped like a diamond. At the back of the head another soft spot is shaped like a "Y."
MOVEMENT	The head will begin to settle into the birth canal toward the end of the pregnancy. There is less movement now because the baby is so confined.

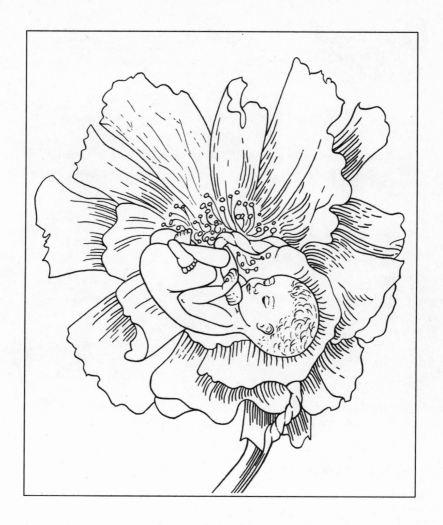

*"The life
which everyone knows
is this momentary period of
the soul's captivity."* [22]

1. Lewis, Samuel, a.k.a. Sufi Ahmad Murad Chisti. *Commentary on Education*, Chapter 3, p. 4.

2. Anonymous

3. Jung, C.G. *Mandala Symbolism*, translated by R. F. C. Hull, extracted from "Archetypes and the Collective Unconscious," Vol. 9, Part I, Collected Works. (P/B #266)

4. Khan, Hazrat Inayat. "Aphorisms," *The Complete Sayings of Hazrat Inayat Khan*. New Lebanon, N.Y.: Sufi Order Publications, 1978, p. 200.

5. Vera J. Corda.

6. Khan. "Salat" prayer, *Complete Sayings*, p. 55.

7. Ibid., "Alankaras," p. 92.

8. Ibid., p. 83.

9. Ibid., "Boulas," p. 19.

10. Ibid., "Nirtan," p. 155.

11. Verny, Thomas, and John Kelly. *Secret Life of the Unborn Child*. New York: Dell Publishing Co., 1982.

12. Ibid.

13. Khan, Hazrat Inayat. *The Soul Whence and Whither*. New Lebanon, N.Y.: Sufi Order Publications, 1977.

14. Khan, "Aphorisms," *Complete Sayings*, p. 195.

15. Verny and Kelly, *Secret Life*, 1982.

16. Ibid.

17. Ibid., "Ragas," p. 105.

18. Khan, "Saum" prayer, *Complete Sayings*, p. 54.

19. Ibid., "Alankaras," p. 91.

20. Ibid., "Aphorisms," p. 190.

21. Ibid. "Tanas," p. 75.

22. Ibid., "Aphorisms," p. 199.

CHAPTER SIX

Birthing Decisions and Health Matters

An early decision as to where the birth should take place and what type of birth experience the couple desires will diminish frenzied activity and allow the mother to gradually attune to the child's developing neuromuscular system. This will also help her to avoid anxiety and stress. The first part of making this decision is to research the many alternatives in birthing that are available today: waterbirth, home birth, birthroom, or hospital birth — realizing that there are disadvantages and advantages to all the alternatives.[1] Choosing the kind of birth experience the couple wants is an extremely personal decision. As soon as the pregnancy is confirmed, the couple should set aside several days to make this decision, writing down pros and cons and their priorities. Just as complications occur that may require emergency hospitalization during home births, so do complications and inhumanities from hospital intervention. Whatever the decision, the woman should totally trust the obstetrician or midwife she chooses.

Couples choosing a home birth should be well-informed about what to do in case of serious complications and should realize that they may need hospital backup in such cases. The modern woman who sees herself as a self-mastered being who does not need hospital assistance should accept that the hospital can be a crucial backup, particularly in unusual circumstances, when emergencies and infant abnormalities occur, and transfusions or other hospital procedures may be necessary.

The couple may also want to write out a list of points to clarify with hospital personnel should an emergency hospitalization be unavoidable.

Couples choosing a hospital birth should realize that many aspects of standard hospital procedure are inconsistent with the sensitivity of the human newborn infant. Such aspects totally disregard the importance of mother, father, and infant spending a lengthy quiet time together immediately following the birth so that they may form lasting ties with one another. The couple can question many commonly used hospital routines and can request that they be omitted at their birthing. Gentle handling of the infant, no slapping, time for bonding, father being present at the birth, and no drugs or anesthetics have been proven to be advantageous for the physical, mental, and psychological welfare of the child. Presenting a written list of the birthing ideals to the doctor can eliminate later evasions of parental wishes. Standing on their religious beliefs, customs, and convictions can often bring hospital staffs and doctors to view things in the parents' way.

Also included on a birth procedures request list could be: whether the cord will be allowed to pulsate before being cut, whether silver nitrate will be dropped into the baby's eyes, whether the father will be able to stay with the mother after birth and whether the father will be allowed to go to the nursery of the infant (or whether the infant will be allowed to room with the mother) in the event of a cesarean section.

The next step for the expectant parents is searching for a midwife and/or obstetrician. This relationship should be established as early as possible in the first trimester. Proper prenatal care is extremely important and the woman will probably wish to make an early commitment to creating a perfect housing for the soul. During the first twenty weeks the fetus is most vulnerable. All the organs and systems of the body are formed during the first two months, and thereafter are perfected and grow in size only. In any case, where virus or rubella is present, amniocentesis should be performed early to ascertain that no harm has been done to the fetus. Early prenatal care from a professional midwife or obstetrician is important because certain difficulties and fears can be averted if they are dealt with early in the pregnancy.

Unfortunately, many obstetricians are giving drugs that are untested and often later prove harmful to the fetus or woman. Most birth defects occur in the first twelve weeks. It has been shown that a three-month-old fetus that normally swims and somersaults actively will cease movements after the mother has been given barbiturates. The placenta passes drugs and medications through its walls to the fetus.[2] It is wise to avoid aspirin, sodium bicarbonate and other antacids, antibiotics, chemical douches or vaginal sprays or deodorants, laxatives, sleeping pills, tranquilizers, alcohol, nicotine, marijuana, amphetamines, cocaine, and heroin.[3] The woman should realize that total abstention from all drugs and medications (prescriptions or over-the-counter products) is the best approach for having a full-term healthy baby.

PURIFICATION FOR HEALTHY BABIES

Purification of the breath is extremely beneficial. Any woman can purify her breath through simple breathing practices in fresh air, by walking briskly in parks and wooded areas and by meditation and concentration on the developing fetus. For the health of her unborn child she will probably want to avoid smoking tobacco or marijuana as well as the atmosphere of smoke-filled rooms, which have the same effect.

Tobacco smoking during pregnancy causes inhibition of an enzyme that helps make hemoglobin, the important factor that carries oxygen to all cells of the body.[4] Smoking when pregnant can be likened to suffocating the fetus. Accumulation of lead in the fetus, a condition that is sometimes responsible for brain damage and later learning disabilities, is another side effect of smoking tobacco while pregnant.[5] Other tobacco-related effects are cardiac defects, high blood pressure in infants, and cancer.[6] Spontaneous abortion is 24 percent higher in smoking mothers than in nonsmoking mothers,[7] and stillbirths and deaths in the first year are 60 percent higher in babies of smoking mothers.[8] In studies of pregnant women, the heartbeat of the fetus markedly changed each time the mother smoked a cigarette.[9] The woman who knows these facts will probably not be able to continue smoking.

Regarding the effect of marijuana smoking on the child, rhesus monkey studies have shown that five marijuana cigarettes per week during pregnancy cause structural changes in the brain of the offspring at sites related to emotions and behavior.[10] In another study, similarly drugged offspring were often hyperactive, aggressive, and lacking concentration skills.[11] It is likely that a well-informed, conscientious mother will quit smoking marijuana during her pregnancy.

Abstention from drugs is a commitment that follows the woman even into the kitchen where she should abstain from coffee, caffeine teas, alcohol, and foods containing preservatives, synthetic colorings, or additives.

Children of women who drink alcohol excessively are likely to be smaller than average at birth, especially in head size, and will likely remain small into adult life, be poorly coordinated, have short attention spans, behavior problems, and heart defects.[12] Alcoholism during pregnancy is known to be a major cause of mental retardation in the United States. If a pregnant woman is alcoholic, she must face up to it for her unborn child's sake and seek help to end her alcohol addiction.

Caffeine is also indicated as a contributing factor to cellular mutations and hereditary changes in bacteria, fruit flies, and human sperm. It is directly linked to spontaneous abortions and coronary problems.[13]

STAYING COMFORTABLE, HEALTHY, AND FIT

Women may experience backaches at any time during the pregnancy. The change in hormones can cause some softening of the spinal and sacroiliac joints. It is therefore important to focus on proper posture; to learn how to lift with the whole body, bending the knees; to keep the feet elevated with a foot-stool when sitting; and to do the classic pregnancy exercises and postures each day to gently stretch muscles and develop good posture. Books or classes on yoga or body conditioning for pregnant women give detailed instructions on such exercises as the squat, the tailor pose, and the pelvic rock, which relieves backache, strengthens muscles for birth, and prevents swayback.

Some of the following discomforts may also be expected, particularly during the first trimester: dizziness, fainting, light-headedness, nausea, vomiting, and fatigue. (Men often wonder why their wives are sleeping so much.) Nausea and vomiting are thought to be caused by a lack of B vitamins, so taking extra nutritional or brewer's yeast, wheat germ, or B-complex vitamins may help. If the woman arises with a queasy stomach, a few crackers while resting in bed may help. This rest could be followed with a light breakfast and high-protein meals the rest of the day. Dizziness is caused by the growing uterus putting pressure on abdominal vessels and vascular changes, such as decreased blood sugar and increased blood volume, which will have doubled by the end of the pregnancy. This volume of blood supplies the fetus with adequate food and oxygen. Other typical physical aspects of pregnancy are: frequent urination, temporary cessation or slowing of hair growth (although this delay is often compensated for after birth), and cravings or dislikes for certain food.

As the fetus grows larger, the woman may become constipated due to less physical activity, uterine pressure on the bowels, and hormones that slow down intestinal activity. Drinking more water and prune juice, eating more raw fruits and vegetables, and adding bran to the diet are likely to handle the problem. Gas may become a problem because of decreased intestinal activity. If this is the case, the woman will probably want to avoid foods that she knows cause gas, such as beans or brussels sprouts. So-called "heartburn" may also occur as the enlarging uterus pushes the stomach upward. To ease this condition, the woman can eat smaller meals more frequently and avoid oily, greasy, or spicy foods. Ingesting baking soda or Alka-Seltzer can harm the fetus. Shortness of breath may occur as the growing uterus compresses the diaphragm against the lower part of the lungs. Propping herself up with pillows while resting or sleeping may ease the condition. Leg cramps may periodically occur due to the uterus pressing on blood vessels that go to the legs, from fatigue, lack of calcium in the diet, or from too much phosphorus absorbed from milk products. Stretching gently to improve circulation to the aching part should ease the cramped muscle. Massage and body work are also good therapies.

Toward the end of the pregnancy, hemorrhoids may develop due to the heavy uterus pressing against the lower bowel, lack of exercise, constipation, or avoidance of bowel evacuation when the urge is present. The best treatment is as for constipation. Another potential aid is doing more sets of Kegel exercises, which stimulate circulation in the pelvic area. These exercises are detailed below. The pelvis may ache some, which is not surprising, since the pelvis is actually spreading to prepare for the birth of the child. Pelvic rocking can help.

Kegel exercises can be done no matter where the pregnant woman is or what she is doing. It is a key to an easier birth and a quicker perineal recovery after birth. It may also improve sexual relations after birth. It involves pulling up the pelvic floor as if stopping the flow of urine. At the same time, the sphincter muscles tighten. The pelvic floor is held tense for two to three seconds and then totally relaxed. This exercise should be done every time it is remembered throughout the day. It can be effective to practice this exercise while stopping and starting the flow of urine, though it should not be done with a full bladder.[14]

Another common occurrence toward the end of pregnancy is sleeplessness: it is getting rather crowded in the uterus. Warm milk before bed and practicing relaxation methods can help. Swelling of limbs is normal for many women. Decreasing salt consumption, elevating the legs, and resting more will help the problem. Fluids should not be decreased because they are needed in quantity for the fetus.

Varicose veins may also occur, particularly if the woman's family has the condition. This can be alleviated by avoiding excessive standing and locking of knees, taking walks and swimming to improve circulation, resting with legs elevated, and wearing support hosiery.

Yet another potential problem is gum bleeding. This is caused by hormonal changes that increase plaque and structurally change the teeth. So when tooth extraction is necessary, it is best to schedule it early in the pregnancy. Flossing the teeth improves bleeding gums. Sucking on lemons should be avoided because it causes erosion of the teeth at this time.

Much lower back pain, headaches, and heartburn during pregnancy can be traced to stress. Stress may be due to tight finances or the expectant father trying to get his professional life together before the last trimester. *Moving the nest and upsetting the security of environment following conception is not wise* and can lead to problems in delivery of the baby. In fact, stress has also been linked to abnormalities in the fetus itself. In studying animals' habits, we find that they do not migrate after conception, yet the average American family moves once every four years, whether or not the mother is pregnant.[15]

It is important that the woman closely watch her body signals and notify her midwife or doctor if certain signs occur, namely, vaginal bleeding, excessive swelling or puffiness of fingers or face, severe or continuous headache, dimness or blurring of vision, sharp or continuous abdominal pain, persistent vomiting, chills or fever, pain or burning when urinating, and sudden gush or steady trickle of water from the vagina. Many of these are signs of miscarriage.

Many scientists surmise that as many as one out of five pregnancies end in spontaneous abortion. These "silent" miscarriages take the form of late and heavy periods after unusually long menstrual cycles. Most occur between the seventh and fourteenth weeks when the fetus is just beginning to form. There are now tests to predict miscarriage.[16] Perhaps miscarriages are nature's way of telling us that the bonding between fetus and mother is not happening at this crucial developmental time. Rejection then becomes inevitable, but the mother must not blame herself, for her body is not entirely responsible. Since 50 percent of miscarried fetuses are abnormal, this may be nature's way of preventing abnormal babies. Later miscarriages occurring between the seventeenth and twenty-eighth week are from different causes.

For most women, severe emotional trauma follows a miscarriage. There may be fear, anger, extreme disappointment, feelings of powerlessness, failure, or guilt, either self-imposed or stimulated by well-meaning friends and relatives. The couple should share the pain and express their feelings, remembering that it is all right to feel grief, disbelief, numbness, haziness, anger, or frustration. Chapter One treats the stages of mourning following miscarriage in depth.

In case of serious accident or injury in the first trimester, knowledgeable counseling should be sought and objective medical advice heeded. Once the decision to go on with the pregnancy is made by both parents, they should go forward without fear, relying fully on divine guidance and united concentration toward full participation in the rite of passage called birth. Bringing forth a perfect vehicle for the new soul to inhabit is the goal.

1. Feldman, Sylvia, M.D. *Choices in Childbirth*. New York, Bantam Books, 1980.

2. Liley, Margaret, M.D. Auckland Hospital, New Zealand.

3. *Birth Defects*, pamphlet 9-0029, March of Dimes.

4. "Tobacco smoking during pregnancy causes inhibition of the enzyme, aminolevulinic acid dehydratase (ALAD), which helps red blood cells make hemoglobin. Deposits of lead in the fetus' brain may cause brain damage." Rosen, Mortimer, M.D., Perinatal Clini-

cal Research Center, Cleveland Metropolitan General Hospital, 1977.

5. Veeneklass. *Physician's Bulletin.* Vol. 24, 15 November 1959.

6. Research at Laval University, Quebec, Canada.

7. Taylor, and Madison. *Journal of Obstetrics and Gynecology.* Vol. 73, No. 5, October 1966, p. 42.

8. Samuels, Mike, and Nancy Samuels. *The Well Baby Book.* New York: Summit Books, 1979, p. 43.

9. Liley, Margaret, M.D. Auckland Women's Hospital, New Zealand.

10. Heath, Robert, M.D. Psychiatry and Neurology department chairman, Tulane Medical Center, New Orleans.

11. Sassanrath, Ethel, M.D. University of California at Davis, Primate Center Medical School, 1975–1978.

12. *Alcohol.* Pamphlet 9-0165, March of Dimes.

13. Rodale, J.I. *Natural Health and Pregnancy.* Moonachie, N.J.: Pyramid Publications, 1968, pp. 33, 110–113.

14. Noble, Elizabeth. *Essential Exercises for the Childbearing Year.* Boston: Houghton Mifflin, 1976, pp. 35–38.

15. "Legacies of World War II," *U.S. News and World Report,* August 5, 1985.

16. Pizer, Hank, and Christine O. Palinski. *Coping with a Miscarriage.* New York: Dial Press, 1980.

CHAPTER SEVEN

Waterbirthing

The tides of conscious birthing have been moving steadily westward in the eighties. It is not surprising that many spiritually awakened parents in Hawaii have opted for waterbirthing. The warm Pacific Ocean waters, the presence of hunas (healers), and the eruptions of volcanos (which are said to bring the goddess Peile once more in contact with humans) are also conducive to building the intuitive body in expectant mothers. Waterbirth is a rediscovered method of conscious and spiritually present birthing.

The remarkable success of waterbirth in America has probably happened because of parents determined to create a new drug-free atmosphere of peace and natural beauty in which their babies are introduced to our earth plane. The strict policies of our medical profession indirectly encourage expectant parents to take total responsibility for their own waterbirths. By drawing upon their inner guidance and wisdom, as their ancestors had done so wonderfully well, parents have been successfully guided through these births without any negative aftermath.

Michel Odent, M.D., author of *Birth Reborn*, has successfully used underwater birth in tanks resembling hot tubs in well over nine hundred births at a general hospital in Pithiviers, France.[1] He found that the buoyancy, warmth, and lack of gravity in the water element relaxes the mother and reduces her inhibitions and bleeding. These conditions also produce alpha brain wave rhythms, which eliminate fear — the greatest cause of pain — and reduce and shorten labor. Birth happens naturally without intervention of midwife or obstetrician. Birthing directly into a warm water environment eases the stress the amniotic sac meets in the birth canal. The submerged environment enables the baby to move around and unfold into our gravity, light, and air without trauma.[2]

Natives of the South Pacific Islands long ago found that the warm ocean water was the best birthing room nature had to offer. Today we are rediscovering their ancient wisdom. For the past fifty years waterbirthing has been quietly practiced in Russia. Pioneer waterbirther, Igor Charkovsky, a physician at Children's Polytechnic in Moscow, U.S.S.R., feels that waterbirthing is the most perfect of birth methods because it introduces newborns to an environment they have already adapted to during their nine months in utero.[3] He says that fear of the newborn's trying to breathe while underwater is not viable because the infant is signaled to breathe only when air is present. Dr. Charkovsky discovered the presence of the automatic breathing reflex that shuts off the windpipe as soon as water enters the throat, so it is impossible for the infant to drown. All swimming instructors of infants prove this when they introduce underwater swimming first. Dr. Charkovsky discovered that this reflex is present in all infants. He dunks them after they come up for their first breath of air, after the umbilical cord stops pulsing and is cut, in order to keep this reflex operating. He warns, however, that babies can become acidotic and hypoxic if the placenta begins to separate or the umbilical cord ceases to pulsate. Most parents bring the babies to the surface within a few minutes, but in Hawaii infants have been kept underwater for as long as forty-five minutes with no ill effects. No learning disabilities are present by the sixth or seventh year.

Dr. Charkovsky experimented with births in the Black Sea, where his assistants were dolphins. Dolphins possess a very strong biologic field and are mammals of the highest intelligence. He found that in the presence of dolphins humans cease to fear the water element. Legends circulate of dolphins having rescued humans from drowning in the sea just by their presence. In Dr. Charkovsky's experiments dolphins provided an excellent psychic environment in which both mother and babies felt quite at home. Dr. Charkovsky believes that the brain, protected from the force of gravity during waterbirthing, retains its more sensitive functions. He also employs bioenergetic cleansing procedures to clear tensions during labor.

Dr. Odent says, "the right place to give birth would be the right place to make love." The ideal place for natural waterbirth would be in the ocean if you can travel to a place where the waters are unpolluted, secluded, warm, and calm. Such places exist in the Bahamas, New Zealand, and Australia. When that is impossible there are many options within the home. Dr. Odent uses round pools seven feet in diameter and two-and-a-half feet deep. Dr. Charkovsky uses rectangular plexiglass tubs, two feet by six feet — long enough for someone to get into the tub with the mother. In the United States, every kind of tub from wooden horse troughs to steel tubs have been used. Fiberglass hot tubs, bathtubs, and natural hot springs have worked well. Dr. Odent believes that one need not worry about specific matching of the amniotic fluid and uses water right out of the tap. Temperatures range from 95 degrees to 101 degrees. Lower temperatures might shock the mother or infant. Higher temperatures could cause blood to go to the mother's feet, thereby depriving the fetus of oxygen.[4]

HOME WATERBIRTH ENVIRONMENTS

All of the parents in my informal survey created birthing environments that suited their particular needs and preferences. Birthing tubs varied considerably, as the descriptions below demonstrate.

A week before my daughter was born, some friends bought a six-foot-long galvanized horse watering trough for me to birth in. The tank was lined with pillows and foam pads for comfort, including one for back support. This was covered with blue fabric for color and a large sheet of plastic was draped over this. Twine was wrapped around the outer edges and held in place with C-clamps. The tank was filled with water from laundry room hoses and the water temperature was kept at about 100 degrees. Salt was added to simulate the waters of the womb.[5]

Building a birthing tub was too costly for us at the time my third child was due so we bought a child's swimming pool from a department store. It fit perfectly in our living room. We also bought a Paloma water heater and a hot tub thermometer. We were delighted. When labor began in the wee hours of the night, we set everything up. How exciting! [6]

WATERBIRTH EXPERIENCES

The laboring mother may enter a different stage of consciousness, much like the dream state, during advanced labor. Sufi mothers quite naturally use the water breath (in through the nose, out through the mouth) and the wazifa (mantram) *Ya Wahabo*. These practices further reduce inhibitions and relax at an even deeper level. Soft lighting, even semidarkness, increases the level of relaxation and reduces adrenergic secretion. Some have used orange-colored lighting, which simulates the color obtained at the heart chakra in kundalini visualization practices, to ease pain. During this stage of labor mothers often become childlike in their behavior. At this point, verbalizing any mental/emotional block to the midwife and/or mate causes the contractions to become more efficient, less painful, and quicker. Releasing and forgiving old hurts from the mate, which may have been silently held in the heart for a long time, will move labor forward.

The moment of birth is a high point for a mother. Everyone in the room is likely to be engulfed in her euphoric state. Each birth is a highly individual experience. The mother interested in spiritual birthing may have her own favorite practices, chants, and music, which mean something to her state of consciousness. Some combination of these is present in each of the birthing environments below.

Everything about underwater birthing appealed to me; the muffled sounds, the dimmed lighting, and the warmth and fluidity of the water — so similar to the environment of the womb. What a beautiful transition into this earthly plane.

Release! He was out but needed to get his face out of water due to his lowered heartbeat. I put him to my breast and told him how beautiful he was as he suckled and looked at me and his papa. When the cord stopped pulsating we put a tiny quartz crystal on his umbilical cord between his body and the scissors. I sang a favorite Mevlevi zikr (remembrance of God chant) while they cut the cord. Soon after I began to feel the urge to deliver the placenta, which should occur out of the water, so I handed the baby over to his papa who was still in the pool. He gently, lovingly, and ecstatically cradled him in the water with his big hands. Ume, as we named him, floated about for an hour-and-a-half more as his papa bonded to him.

From that day on we would return to the tub with him and he would float peacefully in our hands, often falling asleep. Ume has been a quiet and peaceful baby and we learned that this is a common trait of water babies.

Both of Noa's parents shared their stories of Noa's birth. His mother remembered it this way.

At 4 A.M. I acknowledged that my labor had begun. Given the pattern of my three previous births, delivery could be occurring within the next few hours. We rounded up our birthing team and by 5:30 A.M., all had assembled; we gathered for a group meditation. We were tightly bonded as a group with the angels to guide us and the Divine in our hearts. While the birthing crew filled the tub Howard and I took a walk on the beach, where I did my fire ritual dance to the four directions, the Great Spirit and Mother Earth — gathering strength from all the grandmothers and great-grandmothers who had walked this path before me.

Returning to the house I showered and entered the tub. How can I describe the experience of laboring in the water, floating in the arms of my beloved, drinking coconut water, surrounded by an orange glow of the special lighting for easing contractions, and listening to a subliminal birthing tape especially created for labor! With a totally relaxed body the contractions came and went with ease. Several hours passed.

As the contractions took on more intensity the birthing crew and the children gathered around the tub. Together we chanted and with one mighty push out glided Noa's head into the awaiting hands of his papa — so soft, floating beneath the surface of the water, the cord visible, all ready for the birth of his body. Then whoosh — he was out. He came right to the surface and was lifted to my chest. His eyes were closed, and he was breathing peacefully, softly sleeping. We gently massaged the vernix into his skin and slowly he opened his eyes and greeted us with his first cry. Sweet little Noa, which in Hawaiian means "to be free from any restrictions."

His father experienced it this way.

We entered the tub (the bottom half of a flotation tank) about two hours before Noa was born. I could feel the vibrations of the contractions as the water became a conduit of energy. What an honor to be there waiting to catch our child — to be supporting this creation of love! Then Noa glided forth into my hand, blazing in glory, descending from the mystical heights to engage us all in truth and love. In that moment my heart opened as God revealed Himself once again through my child. Separation fell away and our unity and oneness were unmasked. We fell in love . . . once again we had come home. As our son was bonded to his mother at the breast, we were joined in the tub by our three older children and we all bonded as a family. Again Noa was floated in the water with all the children excited to touch and hold him. The angels sang and we cried with joy, "Welcome Noa, bringer of knowledge through water. Our new teacher has arrived."

Another waterbirth story comes from a mother who is affiliated with the Underwater Birth Exchange in Blairsville, Georgia.

Little tufts of brown hair waved with the motion of the water as the head appeared. Then she emerged. Submerged. She turned around, her eyes looking at us through the water. Little hands reached out as if to say, "Hold me, I've waited so long." She took her first breath about twenty seconds after birth while everyone in the room held theirs. She made little gurgling sounds and looked into my eyes. "Welcome, sweetheart!" The cord continued to pulse, aided by the warmth of the water. Then she submerged back under the water after I blew on her face to get her to hold her breath. The look in her eyes was so trusting. Five times more she was submerged to aid in the transition. Then she was held with just her torso in the water. She held her arms open and appeared content and at home. She turned her head to look around, making connection with everyone in the room, greeting those greeting her, her eyes so wise and knowing. I felt it was she who chose an underwater birth.[7]

Below is an inspiring story from a single mom in Hawaii.

When I told my family that I was going to give birth under water — in a hot tub in my garage — with musical background, flowers hanging from the ceiling and candles lit, they were a little skeptical! My grandmother, who had never before seen a birth, was not fearful and was quite impressed with the idea. My friends helped me to convert my garage into birthing and waiting rooms. The birthing room had rainbow draperies and a rented fiberglass tub. The homey waiting room had couches, tables, lamps, pictures, a cradle, and a rocking chair.

I began labor at 7 A.M. and at 10 A.M. my child's godfather-to-be took me for a walk on the beach. As I walked I breathed the perfume of a bouquet of gardenias and bathed in the warm Pacific ocean, where I felt 2000 pounds lighter. For relaxation I lay on a rubber raft — floating and watching the clouds and the palm trees swaying. As the contractions increased, I returned home, showered, and was massaged by a friend.

By 4 P.M. I took a walk in the park and returned to find my friends arriving. They had me lie on my bed and put crystals on my back and calves. At 6 P.M. they filled the tub from a hose through a water-purification system, then through a Paloma [heater] to heat it to 99 degrees. I spent a few more hours in the tub enjoying the scent of the flower lei hung above it. I then took another walk in the park across the street and opened another 5 centimeters.

Back to the tub! My tape was playing the zikr and "Allah, Allah, Allah Hu," to which I added, "Allah, Allah, I love you." Everybody chanted and I pushed as my baby's head came out. My grandmother felt the soft head with her hand and then, with one more push, out came Jean Baraka's body. He looked up and smiled at me from under the water. After about five seconds, the midwife picked him up and put him on my tummy. He cried for a few seconds. I sat on the edge of the tub. After I coughed the placenta came out. I then walked to the couch where my son was put on my breast and immediately began nursing.

BENEFITS OF WATERBIRTH

Parents, midwives, and nurses who prefer waterbirth seem to agree on the advantages to this method of childbirth. For the mother, waterbirth provides a semi-weightless condition that eases lower-back pressure and the discomfort of her contracting uterus. Tension and, frequently, labored breathing dissipate as the warm water soothes the birthing mom. Physical comfort and warmth promote a natural unfolding and cervical opening. Warm water seems to slow the actual expulsion of the baby, allowing perineal tissue more time to stretch, but actual labor seems to progress at a faster rate (after five-centimeter dilation) in the water.

There are also many positive effects for the newborn. The shock of being squeezed through the birth canal is reduced by the close matching of the water temperature with that of the womb. The traumatic environmental shock of gravity and air are also reduced, allowing the baby to stretch out in a relaxed manner, surrounded by warmth and fluidity. Underwater birth allows the baby to relax and ease into the world of sensation slower, perhaps also gaining a better understanding of leaving the womb. A Hawaiian midwife suggested that babies allowed to ease into the world by waterbirth seem to avoid the habit of tension in adapting to new experiences and are therefore able to embrace life more readily and eagerly.

One midwife felt that a waterbirth is contraindicated for a baby whose heartbeat is decelerating dangerously or who shows signs of lack of oxygen (possibly from a compressed cord). She would not recommend waterbirth in situations where it is essential to get oxygen into the lungs as fast as possible.

Midwives and birth attendants seem to feel that their task is made easier in waterbirths because the need for manual counter-pressure on the lower back as well as the need for hot compresses on the perineum are eliminated. Cleanup is easier due to no messy linens.

Descriptions of waterbirths shared by midwives, birth attendants, and waterbirth authors are inspiring and convincing. Here is what they say.

> Advantages to the baby are very apparent in the utterly serene expression of the babies upon their exit from the

womb. Witnessing the utter calm and grace of these wise young beings is truly a miracle. They seem so aware of their surroundings and so content to wriggle free and to squirm, swirl, and spiral their way through the water and then bob to the surface to take their first breath. How nice for the baby to once again be in an environment allowing complete expansion, no more confining walls of a tight, contracting uterus![8]

These babies are like dolphins and seem to develop better coordination, muscular control, and self-confidence from their love of and naturalness in the water element following birth.[9]

Because professional nursing had established in me a traditional, conservative background of birth techniques, I felt apprehensive when I was first exposed to underwater birthing. Much fear surfaced for me and only through the process of relearning and breaking down past conditioning did I come to understand and see the direct positive effects for mother and child during this incredible experience.

You know how good it feels to lie in a warm bathtub when you've been stressed out and hard at work. My experience has shown that a mom usually completes labor within one hour after her first emergence into the water, *regardless if this is her first or third child*.[10]

If a woman labors in water, then has a dry birth, immediately after which the baby returns to the water, the results are quite similar. I like to see all the women I work with in a tub of warm water for labor whether they plan to deliver there or not because the effects are so great.

The gentle nature of a waterbirth experience has a direct effect on the baby's later life. I've seen babies stay in the water an hour after birth, held by their fathers, and it's quite beautiful to watch them unfold on all levels. It seems to be so apparent that since we are mostly made up of water and the baby floats in amniotic fluid throughout womb life, it would be very natural to be born in water.[11]

1. Odent, Michel, M.D. *Birth Reborn.* Translated by Juliette Levin and Jane Pincus. New York: Pantheon Books, 1986.

2. The first waterbirthing clinic in the United States was the Family Birthing Center in Los Angeles, California, operated by Michael Rosenthal, M.D. Since January 1985, 25 percent of the women using the clinic have opted for waterbirth.

3. Seidenbladh, Erik. *Water Babies: The Igor Charkovsky Method for Delivery in Water.* Translated by Wendy Croton. New York: St. Martin Press, 1982.

4. Dr. Odent's statistics on the first hundred underwater births at his hospital showed that the mothers were unscreened for risk factors and were 19 to 43 years of age. Their babies weighed from 4.7 to 9.7 pounds and there were no perinatal deaths. All presentations were cephalic and no episiotomies were performed. Although there were 29 first-degree tears, no infections were present. Dr. Odent's conclusion was that there was no risk to underwater birth. No drugs or intervention in natural parturition occurred. Dr. Odent does not deliver the placenta in water because of the possibility of water embolism.

5. Taylor, Manjula Nancy. Underwater Birth Exchange, Route 4, Box 4636, Blairsville, GA 30512.

6. Zeilah, A. B. Binstock; Maui, 1985. Personal correspondence.

7. Taylor, Manjula Nancy. *Underwater Birth Exchange Parents Bulletin,* Vol. 51, No. 2, 1986.

8. Garzero, Christina. Maui midwife: personal correspondence.

9. Seidenbladh, Eric. *Water Babies.*

10. The mother should be at least 4–5 centimeters dilated before entering the water. Water temperature should be between 97 and 100 degrees. — Merrily Daly, R.N., birth consultant; Maui, Hawaii: personal correspondence.

11. Ibid.

CHAPTER EIGHT

Birth in Our Society

The soul is negative, fully responsive, and susceptible to every influence; and the first impression that falls on a soul takes root in it.

— *Hazrat Inayat Khan*

In the past decade, many natural birthing centers have opened in hospitals because people have been questioning traditional hospital birthing methods in the United States. Many people today who seek a middle ground (and who do not feel entirely comfortable giving birth at home) prefer birthing centers where emergency backup is available if necessary, but the focus is on using natural birthing methods and carrying out parental wishes in as pleasant an atmosphere as possible.

The emergence of birthing centers takes on greater meaning when the standard European birth is compared with the standard American birth. In Europe, more than half of all births took place at home in 1975, but in the United States, 98 percent were hospital births. Furthermore, the infant mortality and morbidity rates in Europe are not as high as ours, even though most of our births are in hospitals with the newest technological paraphernalia. The reason for this striking difference may be the long-standing traditions in Europe that give families a sense of security around birthing combined with an extremely strong focus on excellent prenatal care. In the United States, there is often little tradition or support from the extended family; perhaps the mortality and morbidity rates are a statistical indication of the role that emotions and the sense of security play in birthing.

In the Western world, until very recently, the medical attitude in hospitals seemed to be to treat the birth of a baby as if it were an illness or an operation. Certainly, the escalating trend of cesarean births is more than a purely physiological matter; women had been having vaginal births for millenia before cesareans became popular.

There is an element of fear associated with illness in our society where birth is treated as an illness; there is a tendency to associate fear with pregnancy, which can extend into the confidence a mother feels in her mothering ability. It is also the reason for many frightened and insecure mothers in America who have their children in infancy and toddler daycare centers or who encounter great frustration with their perceived lack of mothering ability at home during the first two-and-a-half years.

When intuition is lost, people turn to books and take courses in child guidance, which, although valuable on one level, often seem to be merely a substitute for what should be an inner understanding handed down by culture and family. As previously mentioned, in older cultures in Europe, Asia, Africa, and South America, we find pregnant mothers being aided by young girls who are often present at the birth. Such customs enable girls to be ready for mothering when their own time comes to give birth.

North American society has largely lost its community perspective; this is reflected in the event of birth often being removed from the society. In older societies, the intense human emotional bonding formed during the birth event was utilized to form bonds within the community as well as within the family. When comparing family life today, in the context of the small, isolated, often single-parent family, with the environment of former generations, where the community was a part of every birthing, it seems imperative to reinstate supportive relationships and nurturing attitudes and customs. In some southern states, everyone in the Sufi community takes part, to some degree, in the birthing. While the labor is going on, the father and friends are attending, and those people who are in the room during the birth seem to be forever bonded to that infant, in whom they have an intense interest and a deep love. There is an expression that they are "sib" with that child in the years that follow. After the birthing, southern fathers often host a communal meal for all to eat.

Festivity has always happened in the older European countries, in South American societies, and among aboriginal people, where the community celebrates the infant's coming into life. In Termoli, Italy, to this day, it is a custom for the entire village to either kiss that baby or to visit the household within the first forty-eight hours after a birth; to congratulate the parents, to bring a small gift, and to be a part of the birthing in some way.[1] This creates a social bonding to the community and enlarges the family, in sharp contrast to the isolated nuclear family in the United States. Here, raising a family is often a lonely occupation because the parents do not have contact with other more experienced caretakers or other young couples. The couple has to face this tremendous challenge alone, whereas when the community shares it, the whole situation is changed or transmuted.

PHYSICAL PREPARATION FOR BIRTH

The mother's health is crucial, as is her diet, relaxation, rest, and positive attitude. The father, too, needs to prepare by giving himself extra rest and freedom in his schedule before and after the birth because the way for the partner to be most helpful in the early months is for him to keep a balanced emotional state.

Last-minute preparations of the baby's room are often hurriedly completed by the expectant father as he reviews his checklist of things to be done for baby. Last-minute touches are frequently added by the expectant mother as she examines once again all the clothing and paraphernalia that friends and relatives have given to her.

A favorable aspect of home birth is the mother's freedom to

arrange the birthing room so that the lighting, colors, direction of the bed, and placement of devotional pictures are to her liking. In this familiar environment filled with the expectant joy of the previous months, she will feel safe and at ease. Being at home, the break in the familiar family routine and diet will be much less severe.

A good home birthing environment should include waterproof sheets, old clean bed linen, a table for the midwife's and/or doctor's case and clean disinfected floors and woodwork. If possible, the room will have been freshly painted by the father. Carpets may need to be removed or rolled back and an old sheet or layers of large sheets of paper placed around the bed to make cleanup more simple afterward. Spiritually oriented parents like to prepare a spiritually oriented environment for welcoming the new soul. This means blessing the room with candlelight, incense, invocation, prayer, flowers, pictures, and draperies. Bringing down the Light and welcoming the presence of angels and archangels brings the divine energy into the birthing room. Ridding the room of old thought-forms and putting up a few pictures of saints or prophets dear to the mother can promote clear points of contemplation. This in turn can encourage the mother's efforts at self-discipline and faith in her ability to keep on top of it. If the couple is planning a hospital or birthing room birth, they should have a checklist of necessary items to be brought.

The couple is advised to make a list of their wishes regarding hospital birth to be discussed with hospital personnel. If the couple is choosing a hospital birth but wishes to have as little interference as possible, the following "I Want" list is suggested.

1. to avoid a perineal shave
2. to avoid induction of labor
3. to allow my partner, coach, and designated friends/relatives into the birthing room
4. to avoid fetal monitoring
5. to have lots of natural juice, water, and ice cubes during labor

6. to avoid pain relievers and intravenous feeding
7. to have the freedom to select the labor and birthing position
8. to have the baby in the labor room, if possible
9. to have a mirror to view the baby's crowning head
10. to avoid an episiotomy, if possible
11. to avoid the use of forceps, if possible
12. to have an attendant take photos
13. to have quiet or music of our choice for the infant when being born
14. to be sure the baby is handled gently during the birthing (avoid holding upside-down, etc.)
15. to have the baby on mother's tummy immediately following birth
16. to assure there is a lengthy undisturbed time for the parents to bond with the infant following the birth
17. to assure that at least one of the parents is present at all times if the baby has to be taken to another room
18. to allow the parents to massage the vernix, if present, into the infant's skin
19. to have a tub full of warm water ready for a Leboyer bath
20. to have candles and incense burning after the birth
21. to allow the mother to see her placenta and possibly to be allowed to take it home
22. to allow the father to cut the cord
23. to avoid the use of silver nitrate
24. to provide the parents with rooming-in service after the birth
25. to allow the couple to go home as soon as they choose.

MENTAL/EMOTIONAL PREPARATION FOR BIRTH

One of the most valuable people at the birth will be the obstetrician and/or midwife the mother has chosen; his or her philosophy of birthing must be in perfect attunement with the mother's own wishes. When a home birth is planned with a midwife and perhaps a doctor on call, prompt access to a hospital for both infant and mother should be planned. All eventualities should be considered by both parents before the event.

As the due date approaches, the first-time father will probably be quietly checking over those aspects of delivery and birthing problems about which he feels insecure. He might check again with the obstetrician or midwife and establish with the birthing coach what are false labor contractions and what can be considered the real thing. He hopes he can be calm, efficient, and all that his mate will need him to be during the coming labor. For those who are fathering a second or more time, the last weeks are still a period of mulling over what is to be expected of them with the second child entering the family circle.

The mother can do positive affirmations to prepare for a positive birth experience. The following sentences can be repeated aloud three times each day before a mirror.

> I am confident.
> I am relaxed.
> My baby feels my confidence.
> I am resting in preparation for the work to come.
> My baby is changing position, getting ready as it should.
> I will birth without fear.
> I feel the protection of the Divine Mother within me.
> Physically, I am strong.
> Mentally, I am relaxed.
> Emotionally, I am confident.
> Spiritually, I am protected and guided by my guardian angels.
> The birth of my baby will be peaceful, natural, and beautiful.

If parents choose to have a second or later birth at home, they also need to decide whether to allow the first-born child(ren) to be present at the birth. When the child(ren) in question are sufficiently mature emotionally and are not likely to be adversely affected by the mother's travail, some couples feel that witnessing the birth may aid the first child(ren) in accepting the new baby. Others do not feel comfortable about how a sensitive or hyperactive child may react. It really depends upon how "tuned in" and enthusiastic the first child(ren) may feel about the coming event and how confident the mother feels about having them present. When children are too young and not yet questioning where they came from, they may just take one look and back off to a corner to play with a toy, totally tuning out the action taking place. Other families have clearly expressed that being together as a family at the birth has built strong unity and led to total consideration for the needs of the new baby on the part of older children. This family bonding experience is described more fully in the preceding waterbirthing chapter. The transition from the role of baby to that of guardian and helpful big sister or brother can be made easier by inclusion in the birthing event.

The selection of all those with whom the mother wishes to share her birth experience is important because the experience forms bonds that last a lifetime. The mother should always have the privilege of deciding who should be present at her birth. When she is a single parent, she may choose a dear male friend to attune to, accept, and welcome the infant into our world. It is impossible to say how much influence the descending soul who enters the body at the first breath has had in attracting to itself the people who give it the energy it needs in the first hour of life. Many babies make eye contact with all guests present.

It is helpful to arrange to have a trusted, loved person to help around the house just after the birth. The "doula" fills the functions of house companion to the new mother. One definition of this term is "Greek slave"; Elena Rassias, director of The Human Lactation Center, Inc. defines a doula as "the other woman who mothers the mother."

The role of the doula is threefold. First, she must be a trusted friend of the mother and mentally harmonious with the father (when a mother, grandmother, or elder relative is either not available or not attuned to the mother). This enables her to know the mother's way of doing things in her home and to avoid disturbing the father's habit pattern (for those fathers who may need to continue their old habit patterns a bit longer). She can also assure him of his very important role so that the moments of feeling displaced by the infant pass quickly. Her primary purpose is to mother the mother, while doing the more demanding tasks of running the home, such as housecleaning, washing, and cooking. This will enable the new mother to regain her strength, adjust to any breast problems, attune to the infant's nursing habits, recognize her own nourishment needs, and adjust to the reality of the baby in her life. All this calls for peace of mind and a new slate of self-expectancies where time and energy are concerned.

The second function of the doula is to reassure and reinforce the positive caretaking techniques with which the new mother is experimenting. Without advising, the doula may give the example of methods that work from her own wisdom and experience. Her practical function is to supplement the mother, not to substitute for her in those tasks that she enjoys doing herself. While functioning as the helper, the doula must also respect the patterns and customs of that home until the new mother is strong enough — physically, emotionally, and mentally — to take on her full-time role as wife and as guide to her child.

Third, the doula brings routine and harmonious readjustment to a new member's entrance into the family circle. If there are older children in the family, she gives time and attention to them. The new mother may be giving only to the new family member at first. By finding small helpful tasks to include the siblings in the care of mother and baby, the doula helps the children feel important and included in the routines of the nursery (at other than nursing times). In this manner, jealousy and resentment of the new baby's needs can be eased.

My doula could not live in but she came early every morning, always bringing a breakfast goody for my husband and a little gift of beauty from nature to me. Hers was a devout nature and her first concern was to be aware of my insecurities in nursing and caretaking in those first days. The woman whose doula is of the same faith as her own is very fortunate, for she will add her own prayers and concentrations to the mundane duties. Like a mother hen, the woman who served as my doula protected my privacy at nursing times, screened the phone calls, and adroitly maneuvered me to rest when my baby napped. By the time her month was up, I was well-rooted in her schedule of rest and activity in balanced time blocks for myself, and had totally skipped the postpartum blues, despite the stress of a wartime birthing.

Many young women live in different parts of the country from their families and cannot have the ideal doula. Nor can every family afford to hire a doula to take the place of an older relative. In such cases, a close friend who is also expecting might be the answer. It is worthwhile trading hours serving in each other's homes. Living near each other makes it possible to trade services, providing that the deliveries are two or three months apart. If a single or childless married friend lives in another city, she may look forward to coming for the birth and remaining as doula. Fathers in pioneer times and those who are living a wilderness lifestyle today (or who share an exceptionally close relationship and progressive outlook with their wives), have served well as midwives and doulas when another woman was not available.

For many new mothers, getting regular relief from the constant demands of nursing and infant care may also come from support groups. Appreciation, comfort, and encouragement in early nurturing experiences is very important at this time. When no one person is available to help, a phone call can often open doors. Calling churches for aid from members, visiting nurse associations, La Leche League, mental health centers, or childbirth associations may often provide help and/or advice by phone.

Fostering a Positive Attitude Just Before Birth

The many fine books on birthing and pregnancy in bookstores and public libraries have sufficiently informed the expectant parents so that they can intelligently choose the manner of birthing that best suits their particular goals and lifestyle. The couple's early investigation of different methods of birthing now pays off in the security they feel in their chosen method. Those first-trimester decisions about the birthing coach, midwife, and/or obstetrician are confirmed.

By the eighth month or thirty-second week, the parents should be well-prepared for any eventuality. If it is a first child, it will probably be lying head-first in the pelvis, ready to enter the birth canal. If the baby is lying transverse or feet-first, an experienced midwife or physician can often gently massage and turn the baby around. Whether this is a first or fourth baby, by now the parents should have made honest decisions on such eventualities as rhesus incompatibility, small pelvis, prematurity, breech position, or cesarean birth. Women who are in their teens or over the age of thirty-five should definitely have hospital backup — and if a hospital birth, rooming-in, if possible.

When a fetus is normal and the mother has healthy blood, a positive attitude toward her birth, and the support of her mate, a home birth should be a wonderful experience. The couple's study and practice of relaxation techniques by now have probably worked out most fears or tensions that may cause intense childbirth pain. Familiarity with the pioneering work of Grantly Dick-Read is recommended, along with the prophylaxis techniques of Fernand Lamaze in breathing and muscular exercises during labor.[2] Waterbirthing, another relaxing technique, is just becoming known in the United States (see Chapter Seven). A final rehearsal to reinforce the teamwork will further reassure both father and mother.

The last mental clearing should be done before labor begins. If the mother feels anything is disturbing her, preventing an absolutely clear conscience, she should be talk it out with her mate now and resolve it to the greatest possible extent. Hopefully, the couple has previously discussed and accepted any eventuality that might befall their offspring; with no blaming of either's ancestry. The spirit and soul of their child deserves total acceptance and love, whatever the birth may bring.

The intuitive birth coach may need to encourage verbal expression by both partners. The loving reassurance of the mate and his fondling often help to open the birth canal, moving the labor forward. The birth coach attuned to the mother's nature encourages her to walk, to sit in her own position, to squat, or to stand during the natural progression of labor.

During the birth, the love between a father and mother expressed without reserve will make the travail bearable. The father's involvement in monitoring the breath and the labor pains makes him a very integral part of the birthing experience. He spiritually backs up the mother through concentration and prayer, thus affecting the birth environment. The first concern of the father or birth coach is to provide an atmosphere of trust so that the mother may express any physical or emotional discomfort that she feels. Sometimes emotional or long-unexpressed blocks existing between mates delay the birthing process. The mother's wishes to walk, sit in her own favorite birthing position, or get on her feet should be respected.

Positive reinforcements that the partner or coach can remind the mother to say to herself are:

I am relaxed.
My baby feels relaxed.
I am working well with my baby.
I have complete trust in my midwife (partner, doctor).
My baby is doing exactly what it should be doing.
I express my feelings.
My uterus is contracting on its own.
My cervix is dilating normally.
My breathing is perfectly relaxed.
My baby is coming quickly.

UNDERSTANDING THE "NORMAL" BIRTHING PROCESS

Learning about the stages of labor in advance can give an idea of what can be expected and what is considered normal in first or later birthings but each woman should also know that she is a complete universe within herself and she may not fit into any prediction for the norm. The first stage of labor is when the cervix thins out and opens up (dilates), signaling when the baby is in the birth canal. The regular contractions of the uterus will increase in frequency and intensity, reaching a peak and then possibly relaxing. During this relaxation time the mother may wish to practice silence and pull upon the inner strength she has built within her being during the months of waiting.

The contractions will probably occur fifteen to thirty minutes apart and last for forty-five to sixty seconds. This process can normally take from eight to twelve hours in a fast first birth, and from four to five hours or less in later deliveries, although the average first-birth time is twelve to fourteen hours. At the peak, contractions occur three to five minutes apart and last from forty to ninety seconds. The mucous plug and the waters in the amniotic sac may then break, although sometimes the amniotic sac breaks at the last second or must be punctured by the obstetrician or midwife. Dilation of the cervix must reach five fingers, or ten-centimeters width for the baby's head to pass through. This normally takes three to five hours, but in later births it may happen surprisingly fast.

At this stage, contractions will be two to three minutes apart. The birthing mother may find that during this transition between stages one and two she feels irritable and nauseated. Her birth coach can be of great help at this time in aiding her to hold back the urge to bear down before the cervix is fully dilated.

Among Sufi midwives, one practice is used more than any other at this stage: the water breath — regularly inhaling through the nose and exhaling through the mouth. During the first stage of labor no effort is made to control the natural alternation of breath from left to right nostril. Recent research indicates that even if no discipline of breath is practiced by the woman, her breath will alternate as does a pendulum from one nostril to the other according to the emotional reaction she has to her contractions.

In the second stage, the actual delivery of the baby begins. It may last anywhere from fifteen to forty-five minutes for the first birth and may be very short in subsequent births. The water breath in its pure four/four rhythm (in through the nose and out through the mouth) then takes over. Now the mother makes full use of her breathing techniques as the dilated cervix signals for the bearing down to begin. As the baby's head reaches the perineum, the woman may experience a burning sensation. The midwife massages with warm oil and gently stretches the muscle to prevent the necessity of an episiotomy or tearing. The cervix becomes fully dilated to ten centimeters and the mother assumes the birthing posture most comfortable for her.

As the head crowns, the diaphragm is filled by inhaling through the nostrils and exhaling through the mouth in a blow-pant (short puffs of breath). This breath cools the burning sensation of the final stretching of the perineum and allows the head to be delivered slowly and gently without tearing the perineum. After the head is born, the father may turn the shoulders and deliver his own baby if he wishes. The head will then return to its sideways position without help. Gentle pushing by the mother aids in delivering one shoulder and then the other as the father or midwife supports the body.

Depending on her position, the mother may be able to see her baby even before the delivery is complete. If she gives birth lying on her back, with a strategically placed mirror, she can see the baby's head being born. This awesome sight gives her a great psychological uplift. She then pushes the infant out on a strong water breath, as a waterfall powerfully drives water over a lip and into the pool below. The baby descends the birth canal on the fire element; in taking its first breath, inhaling and exhaling the air element, the soul is brought in through the fontanel. The mother's breath automatically becomes etheric as she experiences euphoria with her infant.

The third stage of labor expunges the placenta and may occur from ten to thirty minutes following delivery of the baby. (Some parents wish to save the placenta and plant it beneath the roots of a birthday tree. In this case, it should be wrapped in plastic and frozen as soon as the birth attendants have completed their examination.) Uterine contractions begin the process of returning the uterus to its normal size and position. In hospitals, injections or oral doses are given to force this process, but nursing and massage of the lower belly can speed the process. If hemorrhaging happens, pitocin needs to be given orally or through injection to prevent the mother from losing too much blood.

THE BABY IS BORN

While the newborn baby is lying on the mother's bare stomach, the parents may notice that the skin is covered with vernix, a slick white lubricator, or that the skin is peeling and cracked; that lanugo (fine hair) covers the body, or that the baby is bowlegged or pigeon-toed. Even if the head is misshapen from molding, the ears are sticking out like airplane wings, or the skin is blue, red, or yellow, the mother will see her infant as beautiful. Babies are often born with birthmarks, many of which fade as the child grows older. When a birthmark remains in a prominent position, it is wise to view it as a mark of distinction. Edgar Cayce felt that those with prominent marks on the body had different associations among individuals than did ordinary people.[3]

The baby's air passages must be cleared of mucus immediately. As pulsing in the cord ceases, it is clamped off six inches from the infant; a second clamp is placed three inches from the mother. The cut is made between these two points. If stitches are necessary because an episiotomy was performed or the mother's perineum tore, they are taken while the mother holds the baby on her tummy.

Following the birth the mother should drink fruit juice to raise her blood sugar level. Later a sponge bath or shower (with assistance) will refresh her. Loving embraces given to the mother revitalize her at a time when she is extremely sensitive — both psychologically and physically. This aspect of the mother's psyche is well understood by older societies. Modern hospital deliveries often give little importance to pampering the mother. Someone in attendance should groom the mother by brushing her hair, massaging her arms and feet, and embracing her.

Following the bonding of the new family, the couple may choose to lessen the shock of birth for infants by immersing them in a lukewarm bath, thus enabling them to make a less traumatic entrance into our atmosphere. This gives infants the comforting and familiar association with the water element upon leaving the mother's womb and being thrust into this completely new world of sensation — touch of new textures, feeling of air in the lungs, bright sunlight, and loud ecstatic voices. The smile of relief which settles on the infant's face is moving to watch.[4]

Breastfeeding

Breastfeeding is one of the joys of motherhood — an intimate time of sharing that should always be a relaxing time for both mother and infant. Some babies come in contact with the nipple and immediately begin nursing; others seem to need a little coaxing. If the baby seems disinterested, moving the nipple around in its mouth and expressing a little colostrum will usually start it nursing. Colostrum is the yellowish fluid secreted before the milk comes in that is full of antibodies, which give the child a natural immunity, and that also stimulates the first bowel movements. Because there is a vitamin K deficiency in the child just after birth, this vitamin is routinely given to infants in hospitals; however, it is interesting to note that infants who are nursed right after birth do not have such a deficiency.

If this is the first child, it may take a while before nursing becomes second nature. When the baby is small, nursing while sitting up may be the only position that works because the breasts are usually so full of milk that in other positions they block the baby's nostrils while nursing.

The lying-down posture is good later when the child is bigger. It allows the mother to totally relax or perhaps to take a needed nap along with her infant. When sitting in a chair, a footstool can provide comfort by supporting the leg that supports the arm that holds the baby's head. When nursing in bed, pillows can conveniently support the arms.

Sometimes the mother has no choice in being able to breastfeed her baby. The mother's breasts may be in no physical state to nurse, or the baby may be born with leukemia, or a heart or brain problem. Defective genes may affect the mother's milk. In such cases, it is certainly worth trying to locate a wet nurse with plenty of milk. If this is not possible, a second choice should be a goat's milk formula. The fat globules in goat's milk are already broken down, making it easier to digest. Be certain it is raw, certified milk.

Usually goat's milk is diluted by one part spring water to two parts milk; three teaspoons of lactose (milk sugar) is added to one quart of formula.[5] In my family and among many families today when the baby has been unable to tolerate cow's milk formulas, diluted goat's milk worked well until the third month, when supplements were added. Other formulas recommend sesame, olive, or cod liver oil (which should always be refrigerated to avoid rancidity), as well as 50 to 100 milligrams of liquid vitamin C.[6]

Whichever formula is used, the bottle-fed baby should be held often by the mother to establish eye and hand contact — just as with the breastfed baby. The baby can discern mother's tense or relaxed body muscles whether feeding from the breast or the bottle, so it is important for the mother to cultivate a calm attitude and quiet relaxation techniques, whichever method of feeding she uses. The feel of the mother's skin and her body odor are just as important to the security of the bottle-fed infant as to that of the breast-fed infant.

Building regular feeding times is crucial. When intake of

milk is at the infant's demand, the bowel movements are likely to be regular. Frail infants may need to be fed more frequently to help develop a natural stomach rhythm.

A new mother needs to know what is normal in a new-born's stool. In the first two or three days after birth, meconium stools are normal; they are sticky and greenish-black in color and comprise the waste products accumulated in the last weeks before delivery. The first gray-colored stools are called the meconium plug. Greenish-brown stools indicate that the stools are changing, as the baby adapts to breast-feeding. This may continue for up to two weeks, depending on the baby's own internal rhythm. When nursing is well-established, mustard-yellow stools are normal.

Examining the Newborn for Normalcy

All hospital births require a full examination of the newborn infant, including blood tests to determine if phenylketonuria (PKU), a rare medical handicap, is present. Birth defects, such as cleft palate, clubfoot, and head, spine, hip, and genital abnormalities are also checked for.

Physicians also feel it is necessary to test for certain reflexes because voluntary movements only happen when a baby learns that its primitive instinctual reflexes can fulfill its needs. The Moro reflex is tested for muscle tone. When startled, a newborn will normally draw its arms inward, keep its legs outstretched, and curl its fingers as if ready to clutch something. If one leg at a time responds, there may be a weakness or injury in the other leg muscle.

The walking reflex can be demonstrated by holding the baby upright with the soles of the feet on a flat, hard surface (such as a mattress or a table), then moving the baby forward slowly so that it can perform the walking feat. New fathers love to do this to show off their baby's prowess.

When the bridge of the baby's nose is touched, the eyes blink, demonstrating the blinking reflex. When one side of the infant's cheek is touched, the infant normally reacts by turning in that direction, often toward the nipple. This demonstrates the rooting reflex.

The asymmetric tonic neck reflex is shown when the baby is lying on its back quietly, with head turned to one side and the arm on that side extended. The opposite knee will automatically be bent.

The crossed extension reflex is demonstrated when one of the baby's legs is held in an extended position and the sole of that foot is stroked. This causes the opposite leg to flex, pull toward the body, and then extend. The stepping reflex occurs when the front of the baby's leg contacts the edge of a table, causing the baby to raise its leg and take a step up onto the table. The delay that is observable in the ability of the baby's eyes to follow an object when its head is turned to the left or right is called the doll's-eye reflex.

Whenever any of these reflexes is not present at home births, an observant physician should be consulted. The body's own complex inner universe needs time to develop and coordinate. We can only pray and watch and wait for nerves and muscles to coordinate in good time.

Silver Nitrate Stings Eyes

The practice of dropping silver nitrate in the eyes to prevent gonococcal eye infection is now being challenged, since the solution stings and the swelling normally associated with the eyes of a newborn is actually irritation caused by the silver nitrate. Sometimes the eyes are irritated for weeks, and perhaps this irritation interferes with the baby's ability to see clearly and bond with its mother and father.[7] The drops are given to prevent blindness from gonorrhea contracted from the mother's vagina during birth. In fact, there is time to treat the baby's eyes after birth if an infection develops from gonorrhea.

Women having home births should be aware that there is a possibility of having contracted gonorrhea if she has more than one partner, or if her partner has more than one partner. If a baby has oozy eyes after birth, it should be taken to a physician immediately. Other solutions, such as erythromycin, which do not sting the eyes of the newborn can be given. Contrary to what the couple may be told in the hospital (at least in California), silver nitrate is not the law, but merely recommended.[8] If the couple decides to use silver nitrate drops, they can follow the drops with solutions that irrigate the eyes and ease the stinging.[9]

To Circumcise or Not to Circumcise

New parents of a baby boy will have to decide on whether or not to circumcise him. The best approach for the parents will probably be to treat it as an open debate — do research and try to see the operation in its wider context — and then make a decision. They may want to consult some of the books and articles footnoted below. The feelings of both parents should be in accord before the final decision is made. Surgical removal of the foreskin is supposed to be for the purpose of cleanliness and prevention of later infections, and is a religious rite in Judaism, as well as a tribal ritual among Moslems, Ethiopians, and other African peoples.

If chosen, it is not advisable to perform this surgery until at least twenty-four hours after birth to allow the newborn to stabilize his body temperature and get adjusted to the new atmosphere. However, it is claimed that if the infant is circumcised after the eighth day that vitamin K can then enter the bloodstream to coagulate the blood.[10] Waiting a month or two for the surgery will only interrupt feeding patterns that have finally been firmly established.

A creamy substance, called "smegma," created by the sebaceous gland in the foreskin, seems to be implicated in irritation of the cervix, which may lead to cervical tumors. It has also been rumored that there are fewer cases of cervical cancer in Jewish women because of circumcision of Jewish males. Recent research seems to indicate that this correlation is more likely to be due to other factors, such as mean age of mother when first child is born, nutrition, number of children, and hygiene.[11]

Traditionally, circumcision has been widely accepted in this society as a hygienic procedure; its validity has not been greatly challenged. In the seventies, however, some aspects of circumcision began being heavily questioned. A new development involves understanding the biology and function of the foreskin, for it is permeated with tiny glands that secrete pheromones (chemicals that are particularly odoriferous and biologically response-evoking). Circumcision might possibly have some effect on aggressive behavior, evolutionary dominance, and even mating behavior. Research should provide some interesting social commentary when more endocrine research is pursued.[12]

The practice of circumcision just following birth seems inconsistent with conscious efforts to create a comforting, nurturing birth with as little pain as possible added to the inherently painful birth process. Since it is now realized that infants are acutely sensitive in all of their bodies when they are born, whereas previously it was thought that they did not develop sensitivity until later (and were treated accordingly), subjecting them to the great pain of circumcision at birth seems cruel. At times, however, religious, family, or societal pressure to circumcise is very great and needs to be considered by parents. It is a decision that requires careful consideration.

Cultural Birthing Customs

In some Western cultures, the cord is saved, braided as a bracelet, and dried. The caul (a veil that sometimes covers the baby's face) can be preserved by stretching it over cardboard. Later on it can be covered by glass by the father or closest friend present. In my Dutch family, the caul-veils were considered to prophesy psychic ability as well as to predict any danger to grown children living away from home by the change in color to blue-violet. The placenta, too, is handled ritually in some societies. In some societies, it is cooked and the broth eaten by the mother. Some people plant it in the earth beneath a young tree so that the Earth Mother will remain close to the body of that child throughout life.

1. Shreiber. *Anthologist.* Rutgers University (1974).

2. Read, Grantly Dick. *Childbirth Without Fear; the Original Approach to Natural Childbirth*, 4th rev. ed. New York: Harper & Row, 1972; Fernand Lamaze, *Painless Childbirth: Psycho-prophylactic Method*, trans., L.R. Celestin. New York: Pocket Books, 1972.

3. Cayce, Edgar. *Reading No. 573-IF* (1930).

4. Leboyer, Frederick. *Birth Without Violence*, 1st Amer. ed. New York: Knopf; dist. by Random House, 1975.

5. Airola, Paavo. *Everywoman's Book.* Phoenix: Health Plus Publications, 1982.

6. Dreikurs, Rudolph, M.D. *The Challenge of Parenthood.* New York: E.P. Dutton, 1979.

7. Strabismus. *Journal of Pediatric Ophthalmology*, Vol. 15 No. 3 (May/June 1978) pp. 179–183.

8. Weiner, Rosemary. "The Question of Silver Nitrate," *Mothering Magazine*, #15 (Spring 1980) 60.

9. Hornblass, A. *New York State Journal of Medicine*, 26(11) (October 1976) 1875–78.

10. Airola, Paavo. *Everywoman's Book.*

11. King, Lowell, et al. "Circumcision: rite or rationale, or both?" *Patient Care* (March 15, 1978), p. 74.

12. Garden, Shibui. "Letter to Coevolution Quarterly," *Coevolution Quarterly* (Spring 1981), p. 107.

CHAPTER NINE

Bonding and Birth

When the soul comes into the physical world it receives an offering from the whole universe, and that offering is the body in which to function. It is not offered to the new soul only by the parents, but by the ancestors, by the nation and race into which the soul is born, and by the whole human race. This body is not only an offering of the human race, but is an outcome of something that the whole world has produced for ages, a clay which has been kneaded a thousand times over, a clay which has been prepared so that in its every development it has become more intelligent, more radiant, and more living; a clay which appeared first in the mineral kingdom, which developed in the vegetable kingdom, which then appeared as the animal, and which was finished in the making of that body which is offered to the incoming human soul.

— Hazrat Inayat Khan

At birth the father completes the great mysterious cycle by giving back into the mother's arms the developed seed he planted nine months previously. Every father should be given the opportunity, just following the birth, to make eye contact with his child. In Islam, it is the duty of every father to share this glance. After the eye contact is established, the father places his mouth at the child's left ear and says the first lines of the "Bismillah" — "There is no God, but God." This is the first impress in the ear and the brain of the child at birth. It is considered the man's sacred duty and he is allowed by medical doctors, nurses, and midwives to do it. Then he takes his side by the mother while she has her quiet, one-to-one bonding time with her infant.

This first bonding is based on the pulsing rhythm of muscles and nerves being transferred from the mother's body to the infant. Infants, now physically separate from their mothers, begin to absorb their own fluids, breathe their own oxygen, and rid themselves of carbon dioxide gases. On some level, they may realize that the peculiar vehicle that is their body is working involuntarily.

Surrounding the parents or single mother are those people they dearly love; all share their spiraling euphoric joy as their interest turns toward the infant. The mother may experience revelatory inner perceptions or tastes of ecstasy — certainly great satisfaction. The father often feels relief and an expanding sense of self-esteem, especially when he has supported the mother in her breathing, concentration, and changing emotions. The midwife and birthing guests may have joined in the water element practices and felt the ecstasy of the soul's entrance. Ideally those present quietly leave so that mother, child, and father can share the euphoric state alone in this first meeting.

The infant is held nude to the mother's body during the time of bonding. The mother is interested only in carrying her child to her breast, close to her heart. Most newborns will nurse right away, but if not, this drawing close is instinctive and important bonding. Placing the infant to the mother's breast completes a rite of passage. At first the baby may just lick the nipple, but nursing actually involves a set of complementary behaviors that draw the first guide and offspring together.

When bonding is complete, mothers often have an intuitive, some say psychic, attunement with the physical state of their children that will last throughout their adult life. With eyes wide open and senses alert to the new environment, infants lie skin-to-skin on their mother's abdomen and chest. Their eyes search, then stare wide-open into the eyes of their mother. The bonding process has begun, not with the will but simply with love — eye to eye, heart to heart, soul to soul, light to light.

The mother's fingertips gently trace the contours of the little face, the hands, and the feet. It is such a sacred time that every effort should be made to protect and assure its occurrence. These timeless minutes heighten the mothering instinct and caregiving skill. Such births differ from hospital births where infant and mother are separated in the first hours after birth.

Research shows that early-bonded mothers spend more time in giving love to their babies whereas unbonded mothers spend more time in cleaning bottoms. The bonded infant smiles and laughs more than the late-contact or unbonded infant. Bonded mothers breastfeed longer and have fewer problems with night feeding at three months.

Because of the practice of separating infants from mothers at birth, of putting babies in incubators, and of not following the skin- and eye-contact process previously described, the ability of the infant to focus was overlooked by researchers. It was previously thought that the newborn did not focus its eyes right away and that light and shadows in the room were all it could perceive, but it is now understood that during a very short period of time, the eyes do focus and tremendous sharing is possible in eye contact. Previously, researchers did not realize that bonding was taking place through the eyes.

In hospitals, the baby is often removed from the mother for examination immediately following the birth, which prevents the bonding process. Spiritually oriented parents usually feel strongly that the meeting of souls in the bonding experience should precede all other concerns after breathing begins. If this sharing time cannot be respected, then a concerted effort to maximize the time between mother and infant during the first three days is crucial. For example, modern studies have shown that maternal behavior for one year and possibly longer will be assured if sixteen hours of extra contact between mother and infant (other than the time when the baby is nursing) takes place in the first three days of life.

When the separation of mother and infant is prolonged, as in hospital births, mothers report that they sometimes forget momentarily that they even had a baby or that, although fond of their babies, they think of them as belonging to someone else — the nurse or the physician. The affectional ties may be permanently altered when incubator care is necessary.[1]

> When the infant is physically removed from the mother, instead of effecting a transfer of self-love, she has to detach herself psychically from that part of herself, a process akin to, but not identical with mourning. Selfless mothering of and empathy with the infant depends primarily on the mother's investment in the child of self-love. In caring for the child she cares for a loved part of herself.[2]

Bonding can take place with someone other than the mother if the newborn is given to a midwife, female relative, or the doula to hold.[3] Studies show that observers of the labor and birth are more attached to the child than close friends or relatives who were not present. In the past, including other family or community members in the birth experience ensured to some degree that there would be a dedicated substitute mother (at a time when infant or mother were more likely to die in the birthing process).

In cases where there had been mixups in labeling babies in hospital nurseries, it was found that the mother who had bonded with the wrong infant still was content to keep the first one offered her. The fathers, however, did not agree with this. Long after the baby exchange, the mothers would still express, "That was a lovely baby." Nor is bonding lessened by development and growth, for the person the infant initially bonds to maintains a closeness and a psychic connection even years later.

BIRTH EXPERIENCES

Each birth experience is special and unique. Some different versions are shared below.

Mothers often feel ecstacy at the birth of their child. One

mother's journal entry follows.

> You're here! Safe and sound in limb — breathing on your own. How precious and sweet you look! They tell me that shiny white stuff is vernix. To me it's stardust, sprinkled by guardian angels as they ushered your soul into its body.
>
> A part of myself is lost in your being, little angel. Covered with starshine, you lie, all perfectly in one piece yet a severed part of my self-love. My psyche mourns to lose thee even as eye meets eye in soul embrace.[4]

Birth Story: My Second Child

I awoke during a contraction at 12:45 A.M., December 12. At first I didn't know if these were going to go away as they did the night before. So I tried to sleep between them, but I couldn't. I knew then it was time to get ready.

I got up quietly so that my husband, Sam, could sleep some more. I started a bath, had a hearty snack of vitamin C, calcium, and magnesium with Ovaltine and a gingerbread man. Then I did some walks and chants and woke Sam up at 1:30 to tell him the news.

I took my bath. Contractions were now forty-five seconds to one minute long and irregularly spaced. The bath was so relaxing. I puttered around and cleaned up my sewing stuff and did funny things like packing my suitcase as contractions were not coming any closer or stronger. The doctor was called and then I went to sit with my firstborn, Ariel, and gave her some love vibrations before waking her. Ariel woke up and checked to make sure her candy cane was still there. Then she ran to show our midwife the Christmas tree we had put up. She told me that I was getting the baby — she really knew. The sitter and my first angel left, Ariel happily crinkling her candy cane, in pink "jamas" and yellow hat.

Contractions were now about two minutes apart. Sam loaded the car and me. I realize now that I was in transition.

It was about 3:30 A.M. now. Sam said very little, but every word was precious. He said, "Just like God sings using our voice so He has the baby — so just let Him do it!"

Then as I looked up in the sky, I saw Orion watching over us. I really felt that a great soul was coming through. (Maybe that's who you once were, little baby.) All these things helped during this stage of labor while I experienced chills, trembling, and feeling a little cranky inside with the intense contractions.

Conscious breathing, chanting, and my friend's words got me through. True to tradition, I had a two-and-a-half minute contraction when we arrived at the hospital! We went in and I got prepped gently and efficiently by an aide, a wonderful support. She said that I was all dilated, but somehow I didn't understand. I wasn't thinking clearly. All along I kept thinking that labor was just beginning when in fact it was almost over.

Contractions were long and strong. Chanting "Gopala, Gopala, Devakinandana Gopala" got me along, with Sam reminding me to keep centered.

My doctor arrived, broke my waters and said, "Push!" This was the best part of labor. I pushed and pushed 'til they saw your head. It didn't take long. Then they were bringing me into the delivery room and I still didn't believe it was time for you to come. I kept waiting for the doctor to "give me something." I finally asked and he smiled and said, "Why? With one more push you'll have a baby!"

Then the sparks began to fly — an incredible sensation. I thought my bottom was falling off, and couldn't figure out how to tell the doctor. Then everyone said, "Keep pushing! Come on!" I felt like they were my cheerleaders. The doctor said, "Come on, Nanna. Push that baby out!" And I gave a huge push and they all said, "Look, look!" And you were halfway out; and then another push and there, my beauty, you were. Here, crying, and so beautiful! Ten fingers, ten toes, and thick black hair.

Asaalam aleikum! Welcome to you, little angel!

Birth Story: Cesarean Birth

Cesarean birth is special — for me it created a feeling of deep appreciation that I live in a time and a place where it is possible to birth my baby safely when it could have been a life-or-death situation. Cesareans have gotten a bad name because too many doctors were too quick to do a cesarean, but many cesareans are the only safe way for a birth to occur. Birth is entering the world, by whatever means necessary.

After gearing up for a natural home birth, when faced with the reality of a cesarean, it first brought a lot of disappointment and even a sense of failure. But then I realized that cesarean births involve the same miraculous love as vaginal births.

I was awake for the cesarean birth of my son, Owen Sky. I found out twenty-four hours before his birth that the placenta was covering my cervix and vaginal birth was a very high-risk situation. Fortunately, I had time to prepare myself mentally and physically for the cesarean and to arrange for proper care of myself and my son. I spent the night singing and talking to my baby, telling him that at last I would see his face, that tomorrow he would be in the world.

I discovered that I could request to be awake for the cesarean, to hold my baby right after the birth, to have husband, partner, or friend spend time with the baby while I was in the recovery room, and to have my baby with me as soon as I returned to my room.

I had my baby with me almost constantly and found this to be the best possible cure for almost all my ailments. There were pain and mild contractions as the anesthesia wore off. The doctor and nurse offered pain medications, but I found it possible to avoid them by centering on my baby and the joy of meeting him.

I knew that fasting for the first several days after a ceserean is standard procedure, so I prepared an herbal tea blend of alfalfa, comfrey, fenugreek, and peppermint, which I brought to the hospital to help heal me and fortify my milk. I also brought along some miso and vegetable broth powder to substitute for the salty broth they offer at the hospital, and asked my friends to bring fresh juices.

I feel that babies need special care after cesarean deliveries. I was careful not to push for too much, too soon and tried to use this time to just relax and enjoy my baby. We took lots of warm baths and naps together. Nothing was more important than healing well and all my baby needed just then was to be close to me. Later I gradually worked into stretching, yoga, and walks.

Along with the healing of my physical body, my spirit needed some healing. I successfully managed to cope with feelings of guilt, disappointment, and failure by focusing on the facts that I did the very best I could and that my baby and I were well. Vaginal birth after cesarean is definitely possible, so there is nothing to say that I will not, one day, experience a vaginal birth.

It is good for me to share with other mothers who had cesarean births. It is a birth no less magical, special, or wonderful.

UNDERSTANDING DIFFERENT KINDS OF BIRTH

Cesarean Birth

If cesarean birth is necessary, the father alone may need to do the bonding during that crucial and wonderful meeting time after birth. The cesarean mother may have to do her bonding later with her infant at her breast. Some mothers are now able to bond with their infants immediately following cesarean births due to the use of local anesthesia and the persuasive efforts of parents and attendants with sympathetic or understanding hospital operating room staff.

It is interesting to note that cesarean births occur three to four times more often in births attended by electronic fetal monitoring than with those monitored with a stethoscope. An objection to fetal monitoring is that the bag of waters must be broken to attach the electrode to the fetus' scalp. This puncturing causes an instant depression in the fetal heart rate. From my own observation in early childhood education, these babies are more likely to suffer behavioral and developmental problems later in life.

There are postoperative complications in 50 percent of the women delivered by cesarean section and the maternal death rate is twenty-six times greater.

In vaginal births, fluids and secretions are squeezed out of the baby's lungs through the bronchial tubes and out of the mouth by uterine contractions. In cesarean births this does not occur. Consequently, there is a high correlation of hyaline membrane disease with cesarean sections. The rate of cesarean sections in the United States has risen from 4 to 5 percent to 25 to 50 percent.[5]

Premature Infant

When an early birth occurs, parents should know that the weight criteria that sets five-and-a-half pounds as premature is not always accurate — especially in families where small babies are the norm and parents are also small people. "Preemies" need special care because their digestive tracts are often not fully developed nor are their lungs functioning correctly, but they usually catch up later, both physically and mentally.

My grandmother was an infant who weighed less than two pounds on a butter scale and was too small to dress, so she was put in a tobacco box lined with lambs' wool and kept in the warming oven of a great old woodburning stove for many weeks. She was fed from an eyedropper filled with expressed breast milk for many weeks until her sucking reflex developed sufficiently for her to nurse from the breast. While waiting for her child to develop, her mother wet-nursed another child to keep the milk flowing and to nurture her own strong mothering instincts. This fragile premature infant grew up healthy and lived until her seventy-ninth year.

Abnormal Infant

Amniocentesis now enables parents of an abnormally developing fetus to decide to abort or accept the responsibility of caring for a handicapped child all of its life. This responsibility is frequently much harder for males to accept.

The aura of blessing that surrounds birth can however enable the parents to accept any kind of baby they receive, in love and without bitterness, when faced before birth. Spiritually speaking, every physical limitation forces humans to travel a path divinely set for each soul to master in this lifetime. The physical systems of the baby's body predict most accurately the purpose of its life.

Stillborn Infant

Parents today are usually forewarned of stillbirths due to monitoring of fetal life. The emotional trauma to parents cannot be erased by forewarning, but it can be eased by accepting the teaching that the physical housing was not ready to house the spirit and soul of the child. The soul must be strong to make its choice of parents. This strong desire to embody sometimes works against itself, pushing for embodiment before the physical body has attained its proper developmental rhythm.

When some influence disturbs the chemistry of the placenta, it causes the placenta to fail in its task of nourishing. Instead of a certain system or organ continuing to completely develop itself according to its correct timetable, nature simply goes on to the next scheduled development. When vital organs, such as lungs or digestive organs, lose their developmental scheduling, then the housing at birth cannot accommodate the soul.

Only a strong spirit will fight to live despite inadequate organs to function with. After being strengthened on the djinn plane, the same soul will again return to the same mother.

Our whole concept of birth and death must change so that

the grief and personal guilt felt over a stillbirth or an early premature birth is better understood. Just as in gambling, the law of chance is at work. Experts say "things just happen and often we do not know why." No one can be blamed. Viewing life and death as a great cycle of moving into and out of fields of vibration, rather than as final endings can change attitudes. Every birth is a death on another plane. Every death is a birth on another plane. So "death" is our illusion of reality.

If an infant's physical body does not have a mature respiratory system, sometimes it cannot sufficiently attain the breathing rhythm for the incoming soul to enter. Death ensues. Other physical anomalies can also be the cause. Complete honesty of the birthing team and sincere sharing in the grief of parents should be the focus for those in the room. The father seems to suffer most from developmental imperfection, for he frequently sees his child as an extension of himself. Death is a threat to his own immortality. The pain is real.

Allowing time to grieve instead of whisking away the dead body is a must. Saying "good-bye" to the spirit and soul of the baby, sending it home with love, and reassuring it that it will be strengthened and return again is an important ritual for the parents to share. Close friends often tend to avoid the subject and act too embarrassed to discuss it, which makes it even harder for the bereaved couple. In our culture it is the couple who must set the stage by broaching the subject.

It will take time and mutual support to overcome the couple's self-doubts. Understanding and open communication without blaming each other for any traumas during the pregnancy are imperative. Until this experience is fully shared and reexperienced together, the hurt will continue. Taking time to do some purification of the mental, physical, and spiritual bodies before conceiving again is also wise. Separate retreats for grieving couples can release self-blame and reinstate faith in procreating a strong physical accommodation to which the soul can return. Such retreats will enable the parents to renew their hope and faith.

THE SOUL AT BIRTH

Birth is the emergence of body, mind, and soul into a wholly new atmosphere. The first breath of the baby on this plane is death on another plane of existence. Emerging from the waters of its life sustenance, the infant takes its first breath of air, and the soul is embodied on the earth plane, although some souls are embodied hours later.6 It is a most sacred moment. This blessed moment tells all present whether this soul is a gentle or lusty spirit, and whether it objects to our earth plane or welcomes another round of evolution. Newborns are not all the same age at birth. Some souls shine through as "little old men or women" and some seem to be embodying on the earth for the first time.

The energy field spinning over the mother's navel is sucked through the fontanel on the first breath of the infant's physical body, seeming to disperse itself over the head where it forms a pink half-shell light around the head. Surrounding the entire body is an eighth-inch to quarter-inch bluish line, which is the visible innermost aureole of the physical body's electromagnetic energy field. Here it will remain, growing wide when we are "high" and thin when we are in poor health and diminishing entirely at death, as the soul completes another cycle of learning through this life span.

The aureole is not affected by sound, shock, or movement of the fetus as far as one can observe, although it changes with pressure, drugs, and traumatic emotional experiences of the mother such as grief, fright, accident, injury, and virus. In turn, the aureole has an effect upon placenta, amniotic fluid, and the fetus. So it would seem that the physical, mental, emotional, and electromagnetic bodies or fields of manifestation in utero are not altogether inherent in the genetic pattern, the blueprint from which the embryo is created.

During the process of embodiment, the mind is completed and learns distinctions; the mind begins at this point to categorize and separate the angelic Light from the light and shadow of our earth plane. On the earth plane, the spirit learns of emotions as it shows preferences for things, persons, and positions. The spirit also possesses emotions and a power of its own as it drives the soul forward. Young souls manifesting on the earth plane express all they have absorbed from the sphere of the djinn, as the spirit inherits from family and race the physical body it now occupies. Yet the whole universe gives part of itself to the embodiment. "There is nothing in the whole universe which is not to be found in man."[7] For a fuller understanding of soul manifestation, consult the philosophy of Hazrat Inayat Khan and the passage quoted from *The Soul Whence and Whither* at the beginning of this chapter.

Confronted with a whole new environment, the captive soul must immediately function, taking its first bellows-like breath and letting out the first cry of objection. The Sufi point of view is that an infant is an exile from heaven, and that is why the infant's first expression on earth is usually a cry. The five bodies within must be mastered and it must circulate its own blood, digest, eliminate, and regulate its own temperature and glandular system. The body is unwieldy, the head is two-thirds of the height — an inch bigger than the chest, and the arms and legs are half the size of the head. The heart is beating 120 times a minute — twice as fast as its mother's.

On a subconscious level, people remember their births vividly. In various studies, people remembered who was nervous, careless, tired, crying, smiling, or angry, and were able to sense when their father or others were disinterested, afraid, or friendly.

> The view of life that comes out of the mouths of babies is an intriguing and mystical one, of persons in little bodies knowing many things; knowing they cannot yet make their bodies work the way they want and need and who to trust; noting the strange behavior of doctors, the weaknesses of parents, the needs of siblings, and generally learning from everybody and everything.[8]

THE NEW SOUL AND PARENTS LEARN ABOUT EACH OTHER

From the point of initial bonding, the mother's and father's roles separate; the two viewpoints are there from birth. The infant desires food, warmth, and love from the female; from the male, magnetism and regularity of habits. Mothers often see their infants as angels and have absolute trust in that realm of beings. Many fathers' reactions are to mistrust — an attitude characteristic of the djinn plane. Often removed, observant, and almost critical, fathers want to look in their baby's eyes and reassure themselves that their physical development is as it ought to be. The baby's breathing and leg and feet development may worry him. His baby may seem to be such an out-of-proportion being. Later physical development of the infant will reassure him that those now-scrawny legs will one day hold his child upright.

The father usually first checks to see that newborns are all in one piece and physically developed the way he feels they ought to be. Then he may look for the resemblance, the physical extension of himself in the infant. But he also has an innate mistrust of the big leap between the angelic plane and the earth plane. Feet and legs always seem so small and out of proportion.

East Indian Birth Customs

For the first three days, and sometimes for six days after birth, no friends are allowed to enter the room where the child is; only chosen relatives esteemed by the family. They believe that the mind of the newborn is like a photographic plate and the first impression of early childhood makes the foundation for the whole life. In the child, these impressions affect the mind and even the construction of the face and form. The mother also does not appear before friends for the first six days because she is considered to be in that negative state which makes her sensitive to inharmonious and coarse vibrations.

At the birth of a son, beating of drums and gunfire is cel-
ebrated by the Rajput descendants whose dharma (sacred
duty) was warfare. Singing, playing, and dancing gives that
joyous push, like a swing, to commence the child's life on a
forward and upward swing.9

Learning is set in motion with the first sounds the parents
whisper to the infant. Aboriginal mothers and some isolated
South American mothers have a special language that they
speak to the newborn, which may not always be actual words;
it might be cooing, humming, or saying "aaaahh" or "ooohhh."
Some Sufi mothers sing "ishq Allah mahbood lillah" (meaning
God is love, lover, and beloved) or just "Om" soon after birth.
This first tuning, the mysticism of sound, which comes from her
heart and is tuned to her child, also has to do with the initial
bonding. In that first communication the infant echoes "I am
what you give me." What you give your infant in those first
minutes after birth lingers for the rest of the child's life and
foreshadows the emotional security of the adult to come.

The incarnating soul has from preconception dictated how
it would be born, the atmosphere it demands for peace and
tranquility, and how it will enter our earth plane. The Divine
Universal Consciousness has enabled the soul to become both
guide and teacher in utero to the parents. It urges them to get
and stay inwardly clear during the gestation period, integrating
them at the highest possible level of consciousness. This often
means healing their lives by getting in touch with the unconscious emotions of grief, fear, and pain deeply buried from past
losses and bringing the ideal of selfless living for another down
into the ever-new parenting reality. "When we study life
minutely we find that every soul is born with trust, but in most
lives, the original gift of trust becomes diminished, broken,
buried, or almost lost."10 Trust is reborn as each parent gazes
spellbound into the eyes of the newborn, so fresh from the
heavenly spheres. Trust is renewed as the new family unites,
bonds, and begins the new relationship.

Birth is the time when we are closest to the spirit, reliving those hours as on All Saints Day, when we are told the angels are closest to the earth. We become children again, thinking as a child, feeling as a child, being as a child in the presence of a being fresh from heaven. We meet the Being of the newborn as it meets the eyes and auras of the invited friends at the birth, sharing the euphoria of that magic atmosphere and bonding with the soul for a lifetime. The experience opens our hearts, enabling us to hear the Divine Voice as we remember where we came from and where we are going.

1. Rose, E. Furman, and Associates (1960).

2. Kennell, John H., and Rolnick (1960).

3. Mills and Lang (1974).

4. Vera J. Corda, personal journal entries (1943).

5. Mendelsohn, Robert S. *Confessions of a Medical Heretic.* Chicago: Contemporary Books, 1979.

6. Cayce, Edgar. *Reading No. 530-30.*

7. Khan, Hazrat Inayat. *The Soul Whence and Whither.* New Lebanon, N.Y.: Sufi Order Publications, 1977.

8. Chamberlain, David. *Birth and Before: What People Say About Hypnosis.*

9. Khan, Hazrat Inayat. *Gist of Hazrat Inayat Khan.* Series III, Gatha No. 5, "Superstitions, Customs, and Beliefs."

10. Keesing, Elisabeth de Jong-. *Inayat Answers.* London: Fine Books Ltd./East-West Publications, 1977, p. 56.

Recommended Works
on Relevant Topics

WOMEN, CHILDBEARING, PURITY, AND THE SOUL'S DESCENT

Corda, Vera J. *Perfection of Womanhood:* transcripts from workshops. M.K. Fitzgerald, 2451 Road K, Redwood Valley, Calif. 95470.

Ghanananda, Swami. *Women Saints: East and West.* Hollywood, Calif.: Vedanta Press, 1955.

Khan, Dede. *Birth Stories of the Prophets.* London: East-West Publications, 1978.

Khan, Hazrat Inayat. *The Soul Whence and Whither.* New Lebanon, N.Y.: Sufi Order Publications, 1977.

Michael, Arnold. *Blessed Among Women.* Ojai, Calif.: Talking Pines Publications, 1980.

Smith, Margaret. *Rabi'a the Mystic.* San Francisco: Rainbow Bridge, 1977.

Theresa, Mother. *A Gift for God: Mother Theresa Treasury.* New York: Harper & Row, 1985.

ATTUNEMENT TO NATURE

Dillard, Annie. *Pilgrim at Tinkers Creek.* New York: Harper's Magazine Press, 1974.

Russel, Franklin. *Watchers at the Pond.* New York: Knopf, 1961.

Thomas, Lewis. *Lives of a Cell — Notes of a Biology Watcher.* New York: Viking Press, 1974.

NONFICTION: THE FEMININE

Castillejo, Irene Claremont de. *Knowing Woman: A Feminine Psychology.* New York: Viking Press, 1974.

Harding, M. Esther. *The Way of All Women.* New York: Harper Colophon, 1975.

_____. *Women's Mysteries: Ancient and Modern.* Oxford: Holdan, 1976.

Johnson, Robert A. *She.* New York: Harper & Row, 1977.

_____. *He.* New York: Harper & Row, 1977. (This book treats the feminine principle, or anima, in men.)

Lindbergh, Anne Morrow. *Gift from the Sea.* New York: Pantheon, 1978.

Moffet, Mary Jane, and Charlotte Painter. *Revelations — Diaries of Women.* New York: Random House, 1975.

Thoreau, H.D. *Walden: On the Duty of Civil Disobedience.* New York: Macmillan, 1962.

NOVELS: NATURE AND THE FEMININE

Hilton, James. *Lost Horizon.* New York: Pocket, 1984.

Hudson, W.H. *Green Mansions — A Romance of the Tropical Forest.* Cutchogue, New York: Buccaneer, 1982.

BIRTH CONTROL

Garfink, Christine, and Hank Pizer. *New Birth Control Program.* 2d ed., New York: Bantam, 1979.

Shapiro, Howard I. *Birth Control Book.* Avon, 1978.

NUTRITION

Williams, Phyllis. *Nourishing Your Unborn Child; Nutrition and Natural Foods in Pregnancy.* Nash, 1974.

PREGNANCY (EMBRYOLOGICAL AND PHYSIOLOGICAL)

Annis, Linda F. *Child Before Birth*. Ithaca: Cornell University Press, 1978.

Belksie and Dickenson. *Birth Atlas*. 6th ed., New York: Maternity Center Association.

Blechschmidt, E., M.D. *The Stages of Human Development Before Birth*. Philadelphia: Saunders, 1961 (highly technical).

Ellis, Helene. *A Birth Book for My Friends*. Hillsdale, Mich.: Change Rd. Publications.

Gilbert, Margaret. *Biography of the Unborn*. Hefner, 1962.

Hamilton, W.J., et. al. *Human Embryology*. Wilkins & Williams, 1962.

Montague, Ashley. *Life Before Birth*. New American Library.

Nilsson, Lennart. *A Child is Born: The Drama of Life Before Birth*. New York: Delacorte, 1977.

PREGNANCY AND BIRTH (PSYCHOLOGICAL ASPECTS)

Blum, Barbra L., with James L. Fosshage. *Psychological Aspects of Pregnancy, Birthing, and Bonding*. New York: Human Sciences Press, 1980.

Colman, Arthur, and Libby Colman. *Pregnancy: the Psychological Experience*. New York: Bantam, 1977.

Janov, Arthur. *Imprints: The Lifelong Effects of the Birth Experience*. New York: Coward, McCaan, and Geoghegan, 1983.

Verny, Thomas, M.D., and John Kelly. *The Secret Life of the Unborn Child*. Dell Publishing, New York: 1981.

PREGNANCY (GENERAL)

Boston Women's Health Book Collective. *The New Our Bodies, Ourselves*. New York: Simon & Schuster, 1984.

Hartman, Rhonda. *Exercises for True Natural Childbirth*. New York: Harper & Row, 1975.

Elkins, Valmai Howe. *Rights of the Pregnant Parent,* rev. ed. New York: Schocken, 1980.

Maternity Center Association. *Preparing for Childbearing.* New York, 1973.

McCauley, Carole Spearin. *Pregnancy after 35.* New York: E.P. Dutton, 1976.

Noble, Elizabeth. *Essential Exercises for the Childbearing Year.* Boston: Houghton Mifflin, 1976.

Wertz, Richard, and Dorothy Wertz. *Lying-In: A History of Childbirth in America.* New York: Schocken, 1979.

BIRTH

Arms, Suzanne. *Immaculate Deception.* New York: Bantam, 1977.

Berezin, Nancy, et al. *Gentle Birth Book.* New York: Simon & Schuster, 1980.

Bing, Elizabeth. *Six Practical Lessons for an Easier Childbirth,* rev. ed. New York: Bantam, 1977.

Bradley, Robert. *Husband-Coached Childbirth,* 3d ed. New York: Harper & Row, 1981.

Feldman, Silvia. *Choices in Childbirth.* New York: Bantam, 1980.

Hazell, Lester D. *Commonsense Childbirth.* New York: Berkley Publishing Corp., 1981.

Kitzinger, Sheila. *Experience of Childbirth,* 4th rev. ed. New York: Penguin, 1978.

Klaus, Marshall, and Kennell. *Maternal-Infant Bonding.* St. Louis: C.V. Mosby, 1976.

Leboyer, Frederick. *Birth Without Violence.* New York: Alfred A. Knopf, 1975.

Parke, Gray, et al. *Complete Book of Birth.* New York: Simon and Schuster, 1979.

Peterson, Gayle. *Birthing Normally — A Personal Growth Approach to Childbirth.* Berkeley: Mindbody Press, 1981.

Petty, Roy. *Home Birth*. Northbrook, Ill.: Domus, 1979.

BREASTFEEDING

Olds, Sally, and Marvin Eiger. *Complete Book of Breastfeeding*. New York: Bantam, 1973.

MOTHERING, FATHERING, PARENTING

Ashdown-Sharp, Patricia. *A Guide to Pregnancy and Parenthood for Women on Their Own*. New York: Vintage, 1977.

Bittman, Sam, and Sue Rosenberg Zalk. *Expectant Fathers*. New York: Ballantine, 1980.

Daley, Eliot A. *Father Feelings*. New York: Pocket, 1979.

Gresh, Sean. *Becoming a Father: A Handbook for Expectant Fathers*. New York: Butterick Publishing, 1980.

Pierce, Joseph Chilton. *The Magical Child: Rediscovering Nature's Plan for Our Children*. New York: Bantam, 1980.

Schneider, Vimala. *Infant Massage — A Handbook for Loving Parents*. Aurora, Colorado: Vimala Schneider, 1979.

Shedd, Charlie. *The Best Dad is a Good Lover*. Old Tappan, N.J.: Revell, 1977.

Steinberg, David. *Father Journal — Five Years of Awakening to Fatherhood*. Novato, Calif: Times Change Press, 1977.

Index

Omega Press

Other books from Omega Press that may interested you are:

Introducing Spirituality into Counseling and Therapy by Pir Vilayat Inayat Khan

Call of the Dervish by Pir Vilayat Inayat Khan

Mastery Through Accomplishment by Hazrat Inayat Khan

The Art of Personality by Hazrat Inayat Khan

Awakening of the Human Spirit by Hazrat Inayat Khan

Ask your bookseller for these titles or contact Omega Press for our complete catalog, which includes many other fine books and tapes.

Omega Press
P.O. Box 574
Lebanon Springs, NY 12114
518/794-8181

How this book was produced

This book was desktop published on *MS-DOS* personal computers using *Microsoft Word 3.1*. The book was formatted and redesigned by Robin Collier of *Art Support* in Mill Valley, from page layouts by Norman Kanter. Custom *Art Support* drivers generated *Adobe Postscript* files that controlled the output of page numbering, headers and footers, illustration boxes, and double spread pages with registration marks. Final proofing was done on an *Apple LaserWriter Plus* with downloaded fonts. The camera-ready output was produced on a *Linotronic 100* typesetter at *Krishna Copy* in San Francisco and at *Charles Collier Designs* in Berkeley. Illustrations were pasted in. The typefaces are ITC Garamond Light and Light Italic by *Adobe*.